SICK AND TIRED

10 LIFE-CHANGING TACTICS FOR COMBATING SLEEP
DEPRIVATION, SLEEP APNEA, INSOMNIA, AND OTHER
RELATED AILMENTS

MAX SAMPSON

TABLE OF CONTENTS

INTRODUCTION

Since I was a little boy, I've been told that I snore while I sleep. I vividly remember going camping with my class in the fourth grade and being teased the next day for snoring and keeping everyone awake. I hoped that I would grow out of it and that, eventually, my friends wouldn't dread having me over for a sleepover. Unfortunately, hoping that you'll grow out of snoring is like hoping the actress in your favorite movie will one day walk into your local coffee shop looking for you. I didn't grow out of my snoring; instead, it got worse! It got so bad that I was scared that I would end up alone since no one in their right mind would want to marry someone who snores this badly! Luckily, my charming ways and cooking skills paid off, and I managed to land the perfect girl.

After we got married, my wife would often wake me up in the middle of the night, jabbing her fingers in between my ribs. Naturally, I would shoot up and look for something that was wrong. I'd look at her concerned face and ask, "What's wrong?" or "Did you hear anything?" Usually, she would sigh a breath of relief and say, "Sorry, Darling. You stopped breathing. I just wanted to make sure you were okay." At first, I thought she was just being dramatic or sleepy herself, thinking that I stopped breathing when I was actually just in a good deep sleep. However, it came to a point where not only would she wake me multiple times a night, but I would also wake up absolutely exhausted.

Of course, being a stubborn man, I convinced myself that it was normal and that everyone felt this tired. However, when I started falling asleep mid-conversation with my colleague and while driving the car home, I realized that I had a serious problem. I knew that my cousin also struggled with sleeping, so I gave him a call and asked for some advice. I never really knew much about sleep problems or about his condition; I only knew that he slept with a weird space helmet at night. After a brief call, he confirmed that what I was experiencing wasn't normal after all and that I should go and visit a sleep specialist. Eventually, I mustered up the courage and got an appointment for a sleep test.

The sleep test was done at a specific facility where you had to stay overnight. They connected me to a ton of wires and machines and asked me to sleep. After a short interval of sleep, they woke me up with some shocking results. They told me that during the short period of sleep, I stopped breathing 77 times and that I could have died during any of those 77. No wonder my wife was an anxious mess! They then offered me a sleeping mask that covered my entire face. After the initial awkwardness, I got used to it and fell asleep once more. When they tried waking me up, I almost took a swing at the doctor! I was so angry that they woke me up because I had just experienced the best sleep of my life!

Perhaps you're in the same boat as I was a couple of years ago: exhausted and totally depleted, desperate for a good night's sleep. Well, if you are, you're in the right place! If you simply want to learn more about sleep and sleep disorders, don't worry; you're also at the right place. In this book, we'll discuss everything you need to know about sleep, whether you're the one struggling or the one stressed about your spouse. After I got diagnosed, I was determined to help others and not fall into the same stubborn trap as I did, which leads me here. My name is Max, and I am passionate about sleep and general health. I've spent countless hours researching sleep and have spoken to many experts about this specific topic. Let me tell you, there's so much more to sleep than most of us are aware of!

I want to start off by saying, "I get it." I really understand how you're feeling. I get the exhaustion, the disbelief, the brain fog, and the mood swings. I've been there, and I'm happy to let you in on a little secret: You're not going crazy. In fact, you're just sleep-deprived! That's why we need to fix our sleep patterns as soon as possible.

On this journey of sleepiness, we'll learn a lot and discuss many things regarding sleep:

- We'll start by exploring the importance of sleep and how it contributes to our health. We'll look at the science behind sleep and how it places us at risk when we don't sleep enough. We'll also look at the benefits of good sleep and discuss some myths about sleep that need debunking before we can continue.
- Then, we'll look at different sleep disorders and what they entail. The goal is not to diagnose you but to help you see and relate to some of the issues so that you can do something about them.

- Next, we'll look at five life changes that can dramatically improve your sleep hygiene and change your sleep forever (in a good way!).
- We'll also discuss medications that can be useful for sleep disorders and how different medications might affect you.
- If you're not interested in medications, we'll also discuss different treatment plans and devices (like my Darth Vader mask that I sleep with), which can help you significantly.
- Sleep disorders sometimes last a lifetime, so we'll also look at how you can manage sleep disorders over a long period of time and how you don't have to struggle forever.
- We'll look at the role of new advanced strategies and how we can implement these strategies to improve our own health and sleep.
- Finally, we'll end the journey by creating a sleep diary together so that you can start to take action to improve your own sleep.

During the course of this journey, I want to encourage you to take notes or make it as personal as possible. Knowing is only the first step to improving your life. It's in the actual doing where the true value lies. So take it to heart and implement the things you've learned. I will often challenge you with a practical step, and I highly encourage you to commit to these steps and do them. I know firsthand how these practices can be helpful and how important it is to get your sleep sorted out. When you take all of this content to heart and fully commit to it, by the end of the journey, you'll emerge as a brand new version of yourself.

- You'll be able to sleep knowing why it's important.
- You'll wake up feeling energized and ready to face the day.
- You'll be able to manage your moods and feel like your old self again.
- You'll struggle with fewer health-related issues.
- You'll feel confident in your thinking again, able to resist the brain frog and think clearly.
- You'll be able to sleep through the night!

It's not going to be smooth sailing, and the effectiveness of these principles will all depend on your willingness to try new things and incorporate what you've learned. So, are you ready to transform your sleep and become a better, less tired version of yourself? Well, then, let's get right to it! Remember, this is your journey; I'm simply the guide.

1

THE MAGIC OF SLEEP

One of the things I battled with the most was admitting that I struggle with my sleep and that it is actually a big deal. I used to view it as "just sleep," not recognizing the importance of sleep. I used to listen to people as they talked about sleeping "wrong" and thinking that they were completely nuts. It's just sleeping, right? How can you do it wrong? Man, was I wrong! Sleep is a much more delicate matter than we think. Gone are the days of falling asleep underneath the dining table, waiting for our parents to carry us to the car. If only we could still fall asleep as easily as toddlers! Unfortunately, that's not the case, and 30% of the global population over the age of 18 struggles with their sleep (Single Care Team, 2021).

In this chapter, we'll take a closer look at what sleep actually is and rediscover its importance in our lives. We'll look at the science of sleep and what actually happens to your body while you sleep (Hint: It's not just so that you can have weird dreams). We'll also look at different types of sleep and the risk of not sleeping enough hours a night. If you're a regular all-nighter, be warned since you will most likely be challenged not to do that anymore. We'll also look at the benefits of good sleep and how it positively affects your body. Finally, we'll end this chapter by addressing the general sleep myths that everyone seems to believe. It's time to reestablish the importance of sleep and stop viewing it as optional.

Before we jump right in, I want to share with you a quick story. My daughter, Angela, has always been the peacemaker in our home. Whenever someone else was having an argument, she would try to keep the peace and get everyone to get along again. One evening, after putting all the children to bed, my wife and I got into an argument. I can't even remember what the argument was about, but it got heated. After a couple of minutes of back-and-forth bickering, we heard a set of small footsteps walk up to our bedroom door, followed by a polite knock. We opened, ready to hear that someone was sick or had wet the bed. However, instead, we saw little Angela, four years old at the time, with her favorite bunny tucked under her arm. She looked at us, and with dead seriousness, she said, "You two need a nap." We turned to each other, trying not to laugh, and asked her, "Why do you say that, sweetie?" She gave a sigh and started waving her little finger at us, saying, "Because when my friends get angry at each other, my teachers make them have a nap, and then after they wake up, they forget that they were mad."

Even though Angela was incredibly adorable, I didn't take her advice. Only years later, after months of research on sleep hygiene, did I realize just how wise her answer was. It's not that the nap fixes everything, but rather that it's much easier to think clearly, listen effectively, and solve problems when you've had a good night's rest. Little Angela understood the power of sleep much better than we did, and she made sure that we tapped into the magic of it ourselves.

THE SCIENCE OF SLEEP

The first magical element of sleep is the science behind it. Have you ever wondered what actually happens once you fall asleep? I always viewed it as the time when my brain gets to shut down and not do anything. Well, it turns out your brain is actually quite active when you're sleeping and busy with meaningful work. According to Carl Bazil, when your brain doesn't get enough sleep, it won't just be tired when you're awake; it actually won't be able to do what it's supposed to do when you're sleeping, either. When you sleep, your body undergoes a series of events that contribute to your overall health. Your body responds in different ways when you fall asleep, all starting with your breathing. When you fall asleep, your breathing starts to slowdown, which also slows down your heart rate.

Your muscles also start to relax gradually when you fall asleep, and you might even experience muscle paralysis. This keeps you from running around or flapping your arms when you start dreaming. Your eye muscles and your respiratory muscles remain active, helping you to stay alive while the rest of your body relaxes (Suni & Callender, 2020). Your brain activity changes as you go through the different stages of sleep. When you sleep, your brain activity reduces, which enables cognitive repair. You lose consciousness when you're sleeping, and as a result, you have better brain function when you're awake. Your hormones are also quite active when you're sleeping, as they release different hormones to regulate different functions. For example, melatonin helps you sleep deeper and gets released once you fall asleep (Suni & Callender, 2020).

When you don't sleep, none of these processes are set into motion. That's why your body will respond negatively to sleep deprivation. It's not just because your body is *tired* but because there are critical processes that aren't being activated due to your lack of sleep. Different functions get activated during different stages of the sleep process, which is why it's essential that you sleep long enough for all the stages to take place. Let's take a closer look at the different stages of sleep.

Different Stages of Sleep

There are four stages of sleep that your body cycles through while you're sleeping. The cycle doesn't finish once and then wake you up; it occurs multiple times throughout the night. Each stage lasts for a different length of time, varying between 70 and 120 minutes. When you sleep for about seven hours a night, the cycle will repeat four to five times. The four stages consist of three stages of non-REM sleep and one stage of REM sleep.

- **Stage 1:** The first stage is non-REM sleep, which occurs when you fall asleep (Nunez & Lamoreux, 2020). As your body falls asleep and enters a light sleep, your brain waves, eye movements, and heart rate will begin to slowdown. This stage only lasts about 7 minutes and is quickly transformed into Stage 2.

- **Stage 2:** The second stage of non-REM is when you are sleeping lightly. You're not awake anymore, but you're also not yet sleeping deeply. Your body temperature will start to decrease, and your heart, eyes, and body muscles will become more relaxed. The most significant change happens in the brain, with your brain waves spiking and then slowly moving down (Nunez & Lamoreux, 2020). You spend most of your night in this stage of sleep.
- **Stage 3:** The third stage is where your deep sleep begins. You are still in non-REM, but your eyes and muscles are completely relaxed. Your brain waves slowdown even more, and your body gets restorative rest. It's during this stage that cells are repaired, and muscles and tissues recover. If you want to feel rested and energetic in the morning, you need this stage of sleep (Nunez & Lamoreux, 2020).
- **Stage 4:** The final stage is REM sleep, which happens about 90 minutes after you've fallen asleep. Your eyes will start to move quickly from side to side, and your brain waves will increase.

Your heart rate and your breathing also pick up pace, and this is where dreaming takes place.
This stage is essential for processing information and performing more memory functions.

Once the cycle is complete, it will start again, repeating all the stages. Most of your sleeping time is spent in stages one and two, which is why you need to rest for longer hours at a time to achieve the other stages. When you fail to provide your body with enough time to cycle through all the stages multiple times, you will start to experience sleep deprivation, which opens a whole new can of worms. Sleep deprivation can be incredibly dangerous, and it can lead to some severe health risks. Let's take a closer look at what it means to be sleep-deprived and what will happen if you don't get enough sleep.

THE RISKS OF SLEEP DEPRIVATION

Before we look at the signs and dangers of sleep deprivation, let's first establish how much sleep you need. This might vary slightly from person to person since age plays a significant role. However, how much sleep you need remains the same regardless of your lifestyle, habits, or what you think your body is used to. The following hours are suggested by the CDC (Nunez & Lamoreux, 2020).

- 65 years and older: 7 to 8 hours
- 61 to 64 years: 7 to 9 hours
- 18 to 60 years: 7 or more hours
- 13 to 18 years: 8 to 10 hours
- 6 to 12 years: 9 to 12 hours
- 3 to 5 years: 10 to 13 hours, including naps
- 1 to 2 years: 11 to 14 hours, including naps
- 4 to 12 months: 12 to 16 hours, including naps
- birth to 3 months: 14 to 17 hours

The cause of sleep deprivation is simple: it's due to a consistent lack of sleep or a heavily reduced sleep quality (Watson, 2020). Losing sleep once or twice won't affect you too dramatically. However, a constant loss of sleep can trigger some serious problems in your body and mind. Luckily, there are signs of sleep deprivation that we can be on the lookout for to ensure that we get enough quality sleep.

Signs of Sleep Deprivation

When you are sleep-deprived, your body will send you signs and symptoms to alert you that it requires sleep. See these signs almost as a fire alarm, sending warning signs and flashing lights throughout the body in the hopes that someone will respond. Sleep deprivation in adults and children differs slightly, but some of the symptoms are the same. Here are some signs of sleep deprivation in adults that you can be on the lookout for:

- Constant yawning and feeling like your yawning are uncontrollable.
- Dozing off whenever you're not active, like when you're watching TV or trying to read a book.
- Feeling highly groggy in the morning when you wake up.
- Dark circles under your eyes.
- Feeling as if your mind is slow and foggy during the entire day.
- Struggles with concentration and listening.
- Mood changes and extreme irritability.
- Experiencing daytime fatigue.
- Using every free moment you have to sleep.
- Slow reactions and mental alertness.

Just having a cup of coffee or downing an energy drink won't help you stay awake when you're sleep-deprived. The only thing that will help is a good night's rest. In some cases, using stimulants such as caffeine might make sleep deprivation worse and make it harder to fall

asleep (Watson, 2020). With prolonged sleep deprivation, you might also start to experience anxiety, depression, and paranoia. That's because many things happen
in your body when you're sleep-deprived in an attempt
to keep going and keep you alive.

What Happens in the Body When Sleep-Deprived

According to the American Academy of Sleep Medicine, one in three adults suffers from some sort of sleep
deprivation (Marcin, 2015). That means that sleep
deprivation is one of the most common health issues
that we might face. When you don't spend enough time
sleeping, your sexual drive will weaken, your immune
system will crash, and you might even gain weight.
That being said, let's look at everything that happens in
your body when you are sleep-deprived:

- **You Get Sick:** One of the first signs of sleep
  deprivation is that you get sick due to a
  weakened immune system. You might start
  experiencing flu symptoms once sleep
  deprivation sets in.
- **Heart Risk:** Being sleep-deprived is really hard
  on your heart. When you don't get enough
  sleep, you place your heart under tremendous
  stress, which increases your chances of
  developing coronary heart disease.

- **Cancer Alert:** Without enough sleep, your chances of getting cancer increase significantly. Breast cancer, colorectal cancer, and prostate cancer flourish in sleep-deprived bodies.
- **Slow Thinking:** When you are sleep-deprived, your cognitive function will decrease, which makes it harder for you to think. You might struggle to complete a simple task or even make everyday decisions. You might also experience a decrease in your ability to practice problem-solving techniques.
- **Forgetfulness:** Along with slow thinking, sleep deprivation also makes you forgetful. You'll struggle to remember things you've studied or whatever someone told you the day before. You will also struggle to lock in any new information due to a lack of sleep.
- **Low Libido:** When you are sleep-deprived, your libido will disappear. When you sleep for less than 5 hours a night, your sex drive will decrease by as much as 15%.
- **Weight Gain:** Sleep deprivation contributes to weight gain, and it might be one of the biggest reasons why many adults struggle with weight management.
- **Accident-Prone:** When you don't get enough sleep, you are more likely to get into a car

accident. When you drive while sleep-deprived, it's like driving when you're under the influence of alcohol.

- **Bad Skin:** When you don't get enough sleep, your skin will respond with random breakouts and adult acne. You will also get more fine lines and wrinkles, and your skin might even be uneven.

Sleep Deprivation at Different Stages

Being sleep-deprived for an hour or two won't have the same effect as being sleep-deprived for 24 hours. Different things happen in your body when you are sleep-deprived for different durations. Let's look at what happens when you're sleep-deprived for 24 hours, 36 hours, 48 hours, and 72 hours:

Sleep Deprivation at 24 Hours

When you haven't slept for 24 hours, your stress hormones will start to increase in a desperate attempt to fight fatigue and remain alert. Your brain will try to cope without being rejuvenated, which will heighten your stress hormones. Being awake for 24 hours is the equivalent of having 0.1% alcohol in your body. That means you are higher on the intoxication index than those who are allowed to drive. Depending on what you're busy with, this can be incredibly dangerous to you and those around you. A lack of sleep for 24 hours also makes you more likely to recall false memories. You'll be more emotionally reactive and might even experience a decrease in hearing and attention (Theobald & Chai, 2019).

Sleep Deprivation at 36 Hours

At this stage, your health is at risk. You will experience high inflammatory markers in your bloodstream, which can lead to cardiovascular disease. You will also start experiencing high blood pressure due to the lack of sleep. Your hormones will also be affected, causing severe mood swings. You'll basically turn into a grumpy zombie! Your cognitive impairment will get much worse, and you will have serious delayed reaction times. You'll have the inability to concentrate even on simple tasks and won't be able to process social cues. You are also less likely to notice environmental changes, which means your house might be on fire, and you won't notice it (Theobald & Chai, 2019).

Sleep Deprivation at 48 Hours

After 48 hours, you are officially dealing with extreme sleep deprivation. Your body will begin to shut down for microsleeps, which will last 3 to 15 seconds. During those seconds, your brain will shut off completely, even though your eyes might be open. You won't be aware of your surroundings, and you will have no ability to read social cues. You'll be highly irritable and anxious, and paranoia might start to set in. Your memory will become worse and worse, and you won't be able to retain any new information. During this stage, you might also experience hallucinations that cause you to see and hear things that aren't real. Your immune system will also take a massive hit, causing you to produce fewer healthy cells (Theobald & Chai, 2019).

Sleep Deprivation at 72 Hours

When you've been awake for 72 hours, you can expect to have significant concentration deficits as well as a lack of motivation and perception. When you stay awake for this long, you will be in a bad mood, and your heart rate will be significantly higher than usual. You'll feel dysfunctional and miserable since your brain will be fighting against the body's desire to shut down completely. Your emotions will be incredibly fragile, and your mental energy will be drained. You'll experience more and more microsleep moments over longer periods of time. You are more likely to fall asleep while doing another activity, like driving. After 72 hours, paranoia, delusions, and hallucinations will start to increase and take over (Theobald & Chai, 2019).

Now that we understand the side effects of sleep deprivation, it's also necessary to look at the flip side of things. What are the benefits of getting good sleep, and does it really outweigh sleep deprivation's side effects? Well, it sure does! Let's take a look at the benefits of getting good sleep.

BENEFITS OF GOOD SLEEP

Getting a good night's sleep is incredibly beneficial to your overall health and well-being. It boosts your brain power and improves so many other health risks that you might experience due to a lack of sleep. Sleeping is almost like a superpower that all humans have, yet not everyone taps into the power available to them. When you get enough sleep, you will be a better version of yourself, both mentally and physically. Don't believe me? Well, have a look at these ten benefits of getting a good night's rest, and then we'll talk again.

Better Heart Health

When you're sleeping, your body releases hormones that keep your heart and blood vessels healthy. When you already have a heart condition, failing to get enough sleep is incredibly dangerous. If you don't have a heart condition, getting enough sleep can help prevent future heart issues (Stibich, 2021). As we've mentioned earlier, when you go to sleep, your heart rate drops, which allows your heart to take a bit of a break. It's almost like stepping off the treadmill and catching your breath but for your heart. When you sleep enough, your heart will be able to manage your fight-and-flight responses better without putting it in danger (Gallagher, 2021).

Regulated Blood Sugar Levels

When you sleep, your digestive system gets to work. As a result, your metabolism is set into motion to convert food into energy. When you're sleep-deprived, it can cause a lot of problems with your metabolism, which then causes your blood sugar levels to fluctuate (Stibich, 2021). When you get enough sleep, your blood sugar levels will be well regulated, preventing you from developing type 2 diabetes. If your blood sugar levels aren't regulated, you are more likely to experience intense mood swings, low energy levels, and a lack of mental function (Stibich, 2021). By sleeping, you are actively regulating your blood sugar levels to return to normal.

Less Stress

Believe it or not, sleep can decrease your stress levels significantly. Have you ever been worried about something, taken a nap, and then suddenly the problem didn't seem as big? Well, that's because sleep reduces your stress levels (Stibich, 2021). By getting enough sleep, you help your body relax and recover from the stress of the day. When you're stressed, you act in a way that isn't productive or beneficial. You'll start to act out of fear and make decisions that won't help you in the long term. When you get enough quality sleep, you will feel less stressed and be able to manage your feelings and fears better. There are so many things that can cause stress, and we each deal with stress in our own way. However, the more stressed we are, the more we'll feel the side effects. The best way to battle stress naturally is by sleeping and releasing anti-stress hormones (Gallagher, 2021).

Lower Levels of Inflammation

When you're sleeping, your body is restoring your immune system. That means that if there is some inflammation in your body during sleep periods, it is managed and removed. When you have an irregular sleep pattern or don't sleep enough, you will have more inflammation in your body, which can lead to many other illnesses (Stibich, 2021). Chronic inflammation can damage your cell structures and lead to dementia and ulcers. By getting enough sleep, you provide your body with enough energy to strengthen its forces and fight any foreign invaders in your body. That's why the best medicine when you're ill is to sleep it off (Gallagher, 2021).

Healthy Weight

People who get enough sleep are less likely to be over-weight or obese. Poor sleep disrupts your hunger hormones, causing you to eat more and less regularly (Stibich, 2021). The two hunger hormones affected by sleep are ghrelin and leptin. These two hormones are responsible for helping you feel hungry or full. When they aren't working correctly, it can lead to overeating and binge eating. If you want to maintain a healthy weight or lose weight, it's essential that you get enough sleep. Failing to sleep enough will weaken your body, which will cause it to require more energy. Because your body needs more energy, it will prompt you to be hungry more often and increase your appetite. It will also silence the hormone that informs you of fullness, all of which leads to being overweight (Gallagher, 2021).

Better Balance

Have you ever walked and just fell over for no reason? While that might just be a freak accident or due to being clumsy, when you don't get enough sleep, your balance will be weak. You will be more likely to struggle with your physical abilities, which can lead to significant balance problems (Stibich, 2021). This is called postural instability, and it can lead to severe injuries and accidents. When you get enough sleep, your balance will be better, and you will be less likely to be injured by physical activity. That's why it's incredibly important that you get enough sleep if you have a physically demanding job. When you don't get enough sleep, you'll be clumsier and less likely to function physically as you want to.

Increased Alertness

When you get a good night's sleep, you'll be more alert and energized to face the day. You'll be able to focus on the tasks at hand and actually be productive. When you're sleep-deprived, you're less likely to get things done because your body and mind will be too tired to work together. When you get enough sleep, you will feel energized enough to exercise and alert enough to face problems that might occur during the day (Stibich, 2021). When you're able to be engaged in everything you're doing with your day, you'll feel much more satisfied with yourself by the end of the day. As a result, those feelings of happiness and peace will help you have a good night's sleep once again, and so the glorious cycle will continue. When you get enough sleep, you'll have enough energy to keep your mind from wandering away. When you don't sleep enough, you might feel overwhelmed at the slightest inconvenience and be unable to make good decisions (Gallagher, 2021).

Better Memory

While sleep allows your body to recover, it also allows your mind to process information. As you sleep, your brain sorts through all the information in your head and starts filing it accordingly. It empties out short-term memory information and transports the most critical information to the long-term mind (Gallagher, 2021). All of these things enable you to retain information better and remember things from the past. Sleep plays a crucial role in the memory consolidation process, and it enables your brain to link different memories to specific emotions. The deeper sleep you manage to get, the better your memory retention will be. That's why it's critical that you get enough sleep before a big test or an important meeting (Stibich, 2021).

Improved Problem-Solving Abilities

We're all faced with problems on a daily basis. While some problems are minor, others require powerful problem-solving skills. When you get enough sleep, your brain will have the ability to process and understand complex thinking (Stibich, 2021). You'll be better at decision-making, planning, and problem-solving. Getting enough sleep will enable executive function, which is necessary for work, school, and social interactions. If you don't get enough sleep, your executive function will be affected immediately. Making good decisions and being confident in your problem-solving skills will also help you experience less stress (Stibich, 2021).

Healthy Relationships

The final benefit of a good night's sleep that I want to talk about is the fact that good sleep helps you maintain healthy relationships. When you don't get enough sleep, you will be grumpy and much more irritable than usual. It's almost impossible to be in a positive head-space when you don't get enough sleep, making it harder for others to be around you. No one wants to be around someone who is constantly grumpy! How much you sleep will affect your reasoning, language, and communication skills, which are all quite important when building relationships with others (Stibich, 2021). When you get enough sleep, you will be able to maintain good interpersonal relationships that are healthy and thriving.

As you can see, there are many benefits to getting a good night's rest. It's essential that we get enough sleep if we want to be well-rounded, successful people. However, there are a couple of crazy myths about sleep that need addressing before we can continue looking at how to get quality sleep. Are you ready to debunk some crazy myths about sleep? Well, put on your investigator's hat, and let's get straight to it!

DEBUNKING SLEEP MYTHS

There are so many myths out there, especially regarding sleep. Everyone claims to have the answers we're seeking, but in reality, very few people actually promote the truth. Before we look at these myths, it's essential to understand the difference between sleep duration and sleep quality. Some people might sleep for 8 hours every night, but because their quality isn't excellent, they will still be slightly sleep-deprived. On the other hand, if you have good sleep quality, you'll feel rested and energized. Sleep quality can be measured in four ways (Evidation, 2023):

1. Wakefulness: The amount of time that you spend awake after first falling asleep.
2. Sleep Latency: The amount of time it takes to fall asleep at first.
3. Sleep Efficiency: How much time do you spend sleeping while lying in bed.
4. Sleep Waking: How many times do you wake up during the night?

By understanding sleep quality, we're able to look at these myths and identify the mistakes that people make. People often confuse quality with quantity, but that doesn't mean that we shouldn't strive for quantity of sleep as well. Let's have a look at five sleeping myths that many people believe. I also believed some of these myths in my earlier life, so there is no shame if you also believe them.

Myth 1: You Can Train Your Body to Need Less Sleep

Earlier, we looked at how many hours different ages need. Despite that being more or less common knowledge, many people believe that you can train your body to need less sleep. Unfortunately, this is a myth. There's a difference between training your body to need less sleep and just being used to the negative effects of reduced sleep (Newman, 2020). When you sleep for less than six hours a night, you might get used to the effects of sleep deprivation. However, that doesn't mean that your body doesn't still require the right amount of sleep to perform correctly. Without knowing it, you will most likely perform at a lower level, and you'll slowly decline in functioning. That being said, there are a few people who can function for less than 6 hours, but that's due to a specific genetic mutation, not because they've trained their bodies to do so.

Myth 2: Taking Naps Prevents You From Sleeping at Night

I love taking naps during the day. A quick 20-minute nap over lunchtime is all I need to feel energized and ready to face the rest of my schedule. However, I always get snarky comments from others, claiming that my daytime nap will ruin my quality of sleep at night. Well, there's some truth to that, but not entirely. Generally speaking, if you take a prolonged nap during the day, you will struggle to sleep at night due to the simple fact that you won't be tired yet. However, if you are sleep-deprived and can barely function, a quick nap is a great idea and won't influence your sleep at night. When you nap for much longer than 20 minutes, you'll wake up feeling groggy and possibly even more tired than before (Newman, 2020).

Daytime naps are a big part of many other countries that believe in a *siesta*. However, naps aren't only for the sleep-deprived. When you take a quick daytime nap when you're not sleep-deprived, you are more likely to experience subjective and behavioral improvements. Meaning that a nap ultimately makes you a better person. By taking frequent naps, you also lower your risk of cardiovascular dysfunction (Newman, 2020). That being said, we can rest assured that this myth is inaccurate and take our naps in peace.

Myth 3: All Animals Sleep

Since we love sleeping and our hearts melt when we see a puppy or a kitten take a nap, we tend to assume that all animals sleep. Well, according to research, some animals never enter a state of sleep. Sure, they lose consciousness or close their eyes, but they never enter a state of sleep like we do (Newman, 2020). Animals like reptiles, fish, and insects never enter a REM period, so they technically only rest and don't sleep. Sleep isn't just a lack of consciousness but a rhythmic cycle of distinct neutral patterns. According to the authors of the article *Do all animals sleep*, only 50 of the nearly 60 000 vertebrate species can be defined as actually sleeping.

So, this myth is also false. Not all animals sleep, but we're part of the "animals" that do.

Myth 4: The More You Sleep, the Better

Some people have the ability to sleep for a prolonged period of time. I have a friend who can easily sleep until 10 a.m. on a weekend (which means he gets about 12 hours of sleep). I always thought that because of this, he would be super rested and energized, but he always seemed even sleepier than usual over the weekends. Well, that's because the more you sleep isn't necessarily better (Newman, 2020). Longer sleep durations can actually lead to poor health. A study conducted following 276 adults for six years found that those who slept for either longer or shorter periods of time than what was suggested were 27% more likely to develop obesity (Newman, 2020). So, whether you sleep for an extended period of time or for a short period of time, it can be very harmful to your overall health, which means that this myth is not valid.

Myth 5: Sleep Deprivation Can Kill You

This myth is a little bit different from the others. The reason is that there is no record of anyone dying from sleep deprivation. However, sometimes the things that we do when sleep-deprived are the things that can kill us—for example, driving while sleep-deprived or working with heavy machinery when sleep-deprived. So, you won't die from the sleep deprivation itself, but rather from the activity that you do when sleep-deprived. In 1965, a study was conducted where Randy Gardner stayed awake for 11 days and 24 minutes (264.4 hours). Even though he felt terrible and experienced intense symptoms, he didn't die. Eventually, he just passed out and fell asleep (Newman, 2020). So, this myth isn't accurate, but you probably shouldn't test it either unless you're planning on not doing anything while being severely sleep-deprived.

Now that we've covered these myths and looked at the benefits of getting enough sleep, we can move on to the next chapter, where we'll talk about different sleep disorders and look closely at the symptoms of these severe sleep disorders. But first, it's time to create your own sleeping checklist.

MY SLEEPING CHECKLIST

This checklist is for your personal use. It doesn't help us much to have all this new information about how amazing sleep is, but we don't apply it. So, this checklist will help you make the most of your night's sleep. So, whether you want to rewrite it on a separate page or memorize it by heart, use it every night before bed to make sure that you are sleep-ready. These tips will help you sleep better and wake up feeling refreshed:

- Go to bed at the same time every day, even on weekends.
- Stop working on any tasks at least an hour before bedtime.
- Invest in black-out curtains to ensure that your room is dark and cool.
- Skip any caffeinated beverages at least 6 to 8 hours before bedtime.
- Avoid eating big meals before going to bed.

- Exercise every day, but not right before bedtime.
- Create a relaxing bedtime routine to put your mind at ease.
- Use your bed for sleep and sex only.
- Don't drink alcohol for at least three hours before bedtime.
- Move your computer or TV outside of your room and put your phone on timeout as soon as you get into bed.

2

UNDERSTANDING SLEEP DISORDERS

I would like to introduce you to a good friend of mine, Nancy Adler. Nancy is a high school teacher at one of our local schools, and we've been friends for years. She isn't just your average teacher, though. She is one of those teachers who goes above and beyond for her students and often works ridiculous hours to help them reach their potential. She is involved in so many school projects, and she loves every second of it. A couple of years ago, Nancy started struggling to fall asleep at night. Despite being incredibly busy and tired by the time she got to bed; she would simply not fall asleep. So she decided to use that time effectively. Whenever she struggled to fall asleep, she would grab a stack of papers that needed grading or work on one of the other million things she did for the school. What would seem like a good idea at the moment would turn into a nightmare the following day.

Due to very little sleep, she would struggle to stay awake during the day. Eventually, she was extremely exhausted, and she lost her love for teaching. The things that she used to enjoy felt like too much effort, and she no longer wanted to go above and beyond. Eventually, we convinced her to seek help from the experts. Nancy went to a sleep clinic and was diagnosed with sleep apnea and insomnia. With the help of professionals, Nancy was able to treat her sleep disorders and improve her overall health. She started practicing good sleep hygiene, changed a lot of her habits, and started sleeping with a sleep apnea mask. Eventually, Nancy was able to return to her old self and enjoy teaching once again.

Just like in my and Nancy's cases, there are many people out there who are unaware of their sleep disorder simply because they don't know what to look for. Many of us think struggling with sleep is normal when in reality, it really isn't. That's why this chapter is dedicated to understanding sleep disorders and really looking into the different types of sleep disorders and their symptoms. However, sleep disorders aren't something that you can just casually diagnose yourself with.

The goal of this chapter isn't so that you can diagnose yourself but rather to help you see that you might have a sleep disorder and then seek the appropriate help. That being said, I want to encourage you to write down your own symptoms before we start looking at these sleep disorders. That way, you can compare what you're struggling with the different sleep disorder symptoms.

We'll look at insomnia, sleep apnea, narcolepsy, and restless leg syndrome. We'll also look at the connection between sleep disorders and other illnesses.

INSOMNIA

Insomnia is one of those words that everyone uses after one night of not sleeping. However, very few people truly understand what it means to have insomnia. Insomnia is not struggling to sleep once a week due to excitement or too much coffee. It's much more serious than that and shouldn't be treated as "just insomnia." So, if we really want to understand what insomnia is, we need to dive into the medical world and discover what it really means to have insomnia. In this section, we'll look at what insomnia is, the different types of insomnia, how common it is, and the symptoms of insomnia.

What Is Insomnia?

Insomnia is a sleep disorder that makes it hard to fall asleep at night as well as to stay asleep. Insomnia will cause you to wake up early and not be able to get back to sleep. As a result, you'll feel incredibly tired, both physically and mentally. Insomnia can influence your work performance as well as your general quality of life (Mayo Clinic, 2016). Most people experience insomnia to some extent for a short period of time in their lives. Usually, it's due to stress or perhaps a traumatic event. Luckily, there are many ways that we can battle insomnia. For some people, insomnia is only a minor issue, while for others, it can be a significant disruption.

Insomnia will leave you feeling tired and generally ill. You will have trouble remembering certain things, and you might also have a slow response time. You might feel confused and experience mood disruptions like anxiety, depression, and irritability (Cleveland Clinic, 2015). Insomnia can cause you to miss out on the fullness of life and can lead to some serious side effects.

Types of Insomnia

Not all Insomnia is the same. In fact, there are a couple of different types of insomnia that you might be experiencing. There are four main types of insomnia that people struggle with the most. It's important to differentiate between these types since that can help find a solution to insomnia. Let's have a look at the four different types of insomnia (Lamoreux & Raypole, 2022):

- **Acute Insomnia:** Acute insomnia is what most people experience somewhere in their lives. It's when you're experiencing short-term difficulties with your sleep, and it doesn't last longer than a couple of weeks.
- **Chronic Insomnia:** Chronic insomnia refers to insomnia that lasts longer than 3 months and affects your sleep more than three nights a week. This type of insomnia can last a very long time if not treated and can lead to serious side effects.
- **Primary Insomnia:** When you have primary insomnia, it means that your sleep problems aren't linked to any other health issues. Your sleep problems are the primary issue and aren't caused by some other underlying issue.
- **Secondary Insomnia:** Secondary insomnia is the opposite of primary insomnia. It happens when you are struggling with sleep due to another illness. Health conditions like asthma, cancer, and depression might cause insomnia, as might some medications or substance use. In

this case, the insomnia is caused by something else already going on in your life.

The different types of insomnia might determine the severity of the symptoms that you experience, as well as the course of treatment.

How Common Is Insomnia?

Insomnia is actually much more common than many of us might think. In fact, 10% of the world's population experiences insomnia to a certain degree (Cleveland Clinic, 2015). Furthermore, one in every three adults' experiences insomnia symptoms at some point in their lives. However, not all symptoms are medically considered insomnia. Insomnia is classified as one of the most common sleep disorders, yet not many people are aware of it. It's hard to put an exact number on how many people struggle with this sleep disorder since there are a couple of different types. A study conducted by the CDC found that almost 77.9% of high school students suffer from insomnia to some extent. While the majority of people struggle with short-term insomnia, a large majority of adults struggle with chronic insomnia (Gillette, 2023).

Symptoms of Insomnia

Insomnia symptoms vary depending on the type of insomnia. However, there are a couple of symptoms that are applicable to most types of insomnia. Have a closer look at each of these symptoms and note how many correlates with your own symptoms:

- **Difficulty falling asleep at night:** When you suffer from insomnia, you'll find it very difficult to fall asleep at night, despite being tired. Even if you feel exhausted, you'll end up lying in bed, unable to fall asleep. Some people even experience a surge of energy as they are about to get into bed.
- **Waking up during the night:** People who suffer from insomnia will most likely wake up multiple times a night, unable to fall back asleep. You might wake up for unknown reasons or jolt awake due to muscle tension.
- **Waking up too early:** When you have insomnia, you will wake up before your alarm clock, despite being tired. You'll wake up in the early hours of the day, unable to fall back asleep but too tired to get up and start your day.
- **Waking up feeling tired:** Insomnia patients wake up feeling even more tired than they felt the night before. You might want to cancel

plans or not go to work due to feeling extremely fatigued and without any energy. No matter how long you stay in bed, you remain tired.

- **Experiencing daytime tiredness:** Usually, during the day, insomnia patients will experience extreme tiredness and sleepiness. They might find it hard to keep their eyes open, concentrate on their tasks, and hold a conversation due to being so tired. They might be tempted to take a nap.
- **Experiencing irritability, depression, and anxiety:** It's very common to also experience mood disorders with insomnia. Due to a lack of sleep, you'll start to feel irritable, and it can even escalate into depression and anxiety. This can be extremely frustrating for the patient since the mood disorder will further disrupt sleep.
- **Finding it difficult to concentrate and focus:** Due to being fatigued, the insomnia patient will have trouble concentrating and focusing on everyday tasks. You might also find it impossible to focus on even the simplest things and get frustrated with yourself.
- **Increased errors in daily activities:** When you are suffering from insomnia, you'll start to

experience an increase in errors in your daily life. You'll make silly mistakes with activities that you usually find easy, and you might even be too tired to actually care about doing something the right way.

- **Ongoing worries about sleep:** With insomnia, you'll start worrying about your sleep. Since you'll feel exhausted and know that you need sleep, you'll start to experience more and more stress when thinking about sleep, and you might even feel pressure to fall asleep when you're in bed, knowing how terrible you'll feel the next day if you don't get sleep.

As you can see, insomnia isn't something that should be taken lightly, and it can be quite damaging to your overall well-being and health. If you've looked at this list of symptoms and realized that you have checked all the boxes, I highly suggest you reach out to a healthcare professional and get the help you need.

SLEEP APNEA

Since you've already heard my story about my struggles with sleep apnea, you might already have a picture of what sleep apnea is. However, there is more to sleep apnea than just what I experienced. In fact, sleep apnea can be quite a complicated sleep disorder to identify, especially if you live alone. In this section, we'll look at what exactly sleep apnea is, the different types of sleep apnea, how common it is, and the most common symptoms of sleep apnea. Once again, if you suspect that you might be struggling with sleep apnea, be sure to reach out to a healthcare practitioner as soon as possible to get it checked out.

What Is Sleep Apnea?

Sleep apnea is a potentially very dangerous sleep disorder in which you stop breathing while asleep. Your breathing will stop and start while you sleep, and most often, you won't even be aware that it's happening to you (Benisek, 2007). If left untreated, sleep apnea can be incredibly dangerous and can often cause high blood pressure and heart trouble. Different types of sleep apnea occur for different reasons, and they also present with different symptoms. That being said, let's look at the different types of sleep apnea in order to understand this sleep disorder better.

Types of Sleep Apnea

There are three types of sleep apnea, all of which have a different impact on the body. Understanding the different types of sleep apnea is essential in order to accurately determine what sleep disorder you're struggling with:

- **Obstructive sleep apnea (OSA):** OSA is the most common form of sleep apnea. It occurs when the throat muscles block the flow of air to the lungs when they're relaxed, meaning that when you sleep, and your throat relaxes, it starts suffocating you by preventing air from entering your airway and lungs (Mayo Clinic, 2020). Usually, this will result in loud snoring as the air tries to make its way through.
- **Central sleep apnea (CSA):** CSA is less common and occurs when the brain doesn't communicate effectively with the rest of the body. Your brain fails to signal the muscles that control breathing, leaving you without any breath (Mayo Clinic, 2020). CSA is considered a neuromuscular disease, and it's often found in people with heart failure or lung disease.
- **Treatment-emergent central sleep apnea:** This type of sleep apnea is both of the previous types combined. It happens when your throat muscles prevent airflow, and your brain fails to signal the right commands to your body (Mayo Clinic, 2020). This is a very dangerous sleep disorder that requires immediate attention.

All three of these types of sleep apnea require medical attention, and they can be extremely dangerous if left untreated for a long time.

How Common Is Sleep Apnea?

Sleep apnea is uncommon, but it is widespread (Cleveland Clinic, 2015). It can impact anyone, from infants to older adults. Obstructive sleep apnea is more common in specific groups. Sleep apnea is more common in men younger than 50 years of age and in women older than 50 years of age. Generally, people are more likely to develop sleep apnea as they get older and if they are obese. Sleep apnea is also more common in Black, Hispanic, and Asian people (Cleveland Clinic, 2015). Central sleep apnea is more common in people who take opioid pain medications and who are older than 60. It's also more likely to occur in people who live at high altitudes and in people who have atrial fibrillation or heart failure (Cleveland Clinic, 2015).

Symptoms of Sleep Apnea

Some of the symptoms differ between obstructive sleep apnea and central sleep apnea. Let's first look at the symptoms of obstructive sleep apnea:

- **Snoring:** When you suffer from OSA, you are more likely to snore really loudly and constantly. If you have a partner, it might be something they complain about often.

- **Fatigue:** OSA leads to feeling incredibly tired during the day and can result in a sense of fatigue where you're unable to do anything.
- **Restlessness:** When you go to bed, you might experience your legs being restless or feel unable to sit still. You might also constantly feel the need to move while falling asleep.
- **Dry mouth:** When you suffer from OSA, you'll wake up with an extremely dry mouth, and you might also wake up with a sore throat. This is due to sleeping with an open mouth.
- **Waking up gasping:** People with OSA often wake up gasping for air due to a lack of oxygen while sleeping. They might jerk themselves awake multiple times during the night due to a lack of air.
- **Forgetfulness:** Due to tiredness and exhaustion, you'll be very forgetful when you suffer from OSA. You will have trouble concentrating on tasks and will often forget important dates.
- **Depression and anxiety:** OSA can lead to serious mental illnesses such as depression and anxiety. Poor sleep quality can greatly affect

your mood, and you might find yourself more cranky than usual.

- **Constant need to go to the bathroom at night:** People with OSA tend to go to the bathroom more often and have a constant feeling that they need to relieve themselves.
- **Night sweats:** OSA can lead to night sweats and irregular body temperatures.
- **Sexual dysfunction:** When you're suffering from OSA, you might experience a struggle with sexual dysfunction and low libido levels.
- **Headaches:** People with OSA experience a lot of headaches that can sometimes prevent them from going about their day as usual.

Now that we've looked at the symptoms of OSA let's also explore the symptoms of central sleep apnea (CSA):

- **Sluggishness:** People with CSA are often sluggish and feel sleepy, which can be misinterpreted as being lazy or uninterested. However, no amount of sleep helps with the feeling of sluggishness.
- **Poor performance:** When you suffer from CSA, you might also struggle academically.

People with CSA tend to struggle in school and at work.

- **Trouble swallowing:** CSA causes difficulty swallowing, and people with CSA might often experience choking on their food and drinks.
- **Mouth breathing:** People with CSA will breathe using their mouths and not their noses, even when they're awake. They might also experience being out of breath when talking or eating.
- **Sweating:** When you suffer from CSA, you will experience a lot of sweating, especially during the night.
- **Unusual sleeping positions:** People with CSA tend to have awkward sleeping positions, like on their knees or with their neck hyperextended.
- **Bedwetting:** Some people with CSA might experience bedwetting due to losing consciousness when they fall asleep and their brain not sending the right signals to the rest of the body.

Sleep apnea can be very dangerous, and it's essential that you speak to a doctor if you have any of these symptoms. I know it might be scary, but I promise you, it's so worth it! Sleep apnea can be treated, and with improved medical inventions, you no longer have to go to a sleep facility where they keep you overnight. When sleep apnea is left untreated, it can lead to heart problems, diabetes, liver complications, and metabolic syndrome. So, it's best to get it checked out sooner rather than later.

NARCOLEPSY

The next sleep disorder we're looking at is narcolepsy. Narcolepsy is not as well-known as insomnia and sleep apnea, but it can be equally dangerous and disabling. Narcolepsy can significantly affect your daily activities, and in severe cases, it can lead to the patient not being able to do any everyday activities on their own. When left untreated, narcolepsy can lead to psychological, social, and cognitive dysfunction (National Institute of Neurological Disorders and Stroke, 2023). Let's have a look at what narcolepsy really is, the different types of narcolepsy and how common narcolepsy is. We'll also look at the symptoms of narcolepsy.

What Is Narcolepsy?

Narcolepsy is a neurological disorder that affects the brain's ability to control your sleep-wake cycles (National Institute of Neurological Disorders, 2023). In other words, you don't have control over when you sleep or when you're awake. People with narcolepsy often wake up feeling rested and energized for the day but then feel extremely sleepy as soon as they start doing anything. People with narcolepsy experience uneven sleep patterns that are often interrupted by moments of feeling remarkably awake. Narcolepsy can be extremely dangerous since many people fall asleep while busy with something else. For example, they might go limp while driving or fall asleep while eating. When you suffer from narcolepsy, you often have vivid dreams and hallucinations and then experience paralysis before falling asleep (National Institute of Neurological Disorders, 2023).

A normal person will enter REM sleep after about 60 to 90 minutes of sleep, while someone with narcolepsy enters REM sleep within 15 minutes of sleep. This causes you to feel paralyzed and unable to act out your dream accordingly. Narcolepsy can lead to other serious psychological, social, and cognitive disorders when left untreated. Unfortunately, narcolepsy is lifelong, but symptoms can improve with the right treatment.

Types of Narcolepsy

There are mainly two types of narcolepsy, which are referred to as type 1 and type 2. Narcolepsy type 1 (NT1) was formerly known as narcolepsy with cataplexy, which is the sudden loss of muscle tone. However, not everyone with narcolepsy type 1 experiences cataplexy. The narcolepsy type 1 diagnosis is based on the patient's brain hormone called hypocretin. When there is a lack of this hormone, and you experience other narcolepsy symptoms, you'll get this diagnosis (Suni, 2021).

Narcolepsy type 2 has similar symptoms to narcolepsy type 1, but without the lower levels of hypocretin and without cataplexy. A majority of people experience this type of narcolepsy, and in rare cases, narcolepsy type 2 can transform into narcolepsy type 1 (Suni, 2021).

How Common Is Narcolepsy?

Narcolepsy is relatively rare, and it affects around 20 people per 100,000 people in the United States (Suni, 2021). Narcolepsy type 2 is also much more common than type 1. In general, narcolepsy affects both males and females, and symptoms start to show at a very young age. Between the ages of 7 and 27, patients are diagnosed with narcolepsy, but in some cases, it gets misdiagnosed with other conditions. Some people suffer for years before getting a proper diagnosis.

However, it is more common in certain patients who have

- autoimmune disorders
- a family history of narcolepsy
- experienced brain injuries

The cause of narcolepsy depends on many factors, but all are linked to the hypothalamus. The hypothalamus is an area in the brain that regulates sleep and wakefulness (Cleveland Clinic, 2020).

Symptoms of Narcolepsy

There are many symptoms of narcolepsy, and some symptoms appear different in different people. However, there are a couple of symptoms that all people with narcolepsy experience (Suni, 2021). Let's have a closer look at the most common symptoms of narcolepsy:

- **Excessive daytime sleepiness (EDS):** EDS is one of the most prominent symptoms of narcolepsy, and it affects all people with this specific sleeping disorder. When you experience EDS, you will have the irresistible urge to sleep in monotonous situations. You'll often feel drowsy, which can lead to sleep attacks. A sleep attack takes place when you fall asleep without any warning. Usually, after a short nap, someone with narcolepsy will feel temporarily refreshed (Suni, 2021).

- **Automatic behavior:** When you try to avoid sleepiness, your body, and mind might start acting automatically. You might be completely unaware of this behavior, and it might appear to others as if you're paying attention. For example, scribbling lines on a page or writing gibberish instead of taking notes in class (Suni, 2021). To others, it might seem like you are participating, but you are completely unaware of what's happening.
- **Sleep-Related hallucinations:** With narcolepsy, you will experience vivid imagery when you're falling asleep, which is called hypnagogic hallucinations. However, you might also experience these hallucinations when you're awake. These hallucinations are often accompanied by sleep paralysis, which can be quite scary and disturbing (Suni, 2021).
- **Cataplexy:** As mentioned earlier, cataplexy is the sudden loss of muscle control that happens to people who have narcolepsy type 1. Cataplexy is often a response to experiencing certain emotions, like joy and laughter.

Cataplexy can last for several minutes, and for some people, it can occur a dozen times a day (Suni, 2021).

- **Disrupted nighttime sleep:** People with narcolepsy commonly struggle with sleep fragmentation. Sleep fragmentation occurs when you awaken multiple times during the night. Other bothersome sleep problems, like sleep apnea, are also common when you have narcolepsy. In general, you don't get a great night's rest.
- **Sleep paralysis:** Sleep paralysis happens when you are unable to move when you are waking up or falling asleep. It's a very unpleasant experience, and it can lead to a lot of anxiety and mental stress. People with narcolepsy have a higher rate of sleep paralysis than those who don't have narcolepsy.

Narcolepsy is a dangerous sleep disorder that shouldn't be left unaddressed. Since it can be hard to diagnose, it's essential that you take note of your own symptoms and consider whether you might be at risk. I highly recommend talking to your local healthcare provider to address any concerns that you might have. Many people with narcolepsy experience social withdrawal after being diagnosed due to feeling ashamed, so it's essential that you have a sound support system around you and that you are intentional about building and maintaining relationships.

RESTLESS LEGS SYNDROME

Have you ever experienced the inability to keep your body still? For many, that happens when they have a full bladder or experience growing pain, but for others, it's a bit more serious than that. Restless legs syndrome happens when you feel the urge to move your body, especially your legs, preventing you from sleeping or getting comfortable in bed (NHS Inform, 2023). In many cases, restless leg syndrome happens when people are stressed, while other people experience it every day. Restless legs syndrome alone seems fairly harmless, but it can lead to many other severe sleeping disorders. Let's have a look at what exactly restless legs syndrome is, the different types of restless legs syndrome, as well as the symptoms.

What Is Restless Legs Syndrome?

Also known as Willis-Ekbom disease, restless legs syndrome is a common condition of the nervous system that causes an overwhelming urge to move the legs or arms. For most people, symptoms appear in the late afternoon or evening hours and grow more intense at bedtime. This makes it incredibly difficult to fall and stay asleep. Restless legs syndrome symptoms are easily relieved by walking or moving around, but that's not always a possible option. This disorder is both a sleep and a movement disorder, and it usually lasts a lifetime (National Institute of Neurological Disorders, 2023). Restless legs syndrome causes an unpleasant sensation in the feet, calves, and thighs that urges you to move your legs at all times. Most commonly, you start to experience restless legs when you are lying down or sitting for long periods, like when you're driving or in the cinema. While seemingly harmless, restless legs syndrome is incredibly uncomfortable and can affect your sleep health. The causes of restless legs syndrome are unknown, but many believe that it is a genetic disorder.

Other possible causes of restless legs syndrome include

- iron deficiency
- uremia
- depression
- fibromyalgia
- diabetes
- kidney disease
- pregnancy
- parkinsons
- arthritis

Types of Restless Legs Syndrome

There are two types of restless legs syndrome, which are known as primary restless legs syndrome and secondary restless legs syndrome (Mansur et al., 2023). Primary restless legs syndrome affects the central nervous system and is mainly caused by genetics. Secondary restless legs syndrome is caused by other health issues such as celiac disease and peripheral neuropathy. The symptoms of these two types are identical, and the effects that they have on your life are also the same. The only real difference is the assumed cause.

How Common Is Restless Legs Syndrome?

Restless legs syndrome can affect people of any age, including children and teenagers. While some people experience symptoms while they're young, others only start to experience them during adulthood. Restless legs syndrome is more common in women than in men, and up to 10% of the United States population struggles with restless legs syndrome (Cleveland Clinic, 2020a). Restless legs syndrome is very common, and people often fail to acknowledge the severity of this disorder due to symptoms coming and going.

Symptoms of Restless Legs Syndrome

There are many symptoms of restless legs syndrome, and the symptoms for primary and secondary restless legs syndrome are the same. Let's have a look at some of the most common symptoms (Cleveland Clinic, 2020a):

- **Leg discomfort:** This discomfort is often described as creeping, itching, pulling, tugging, burning, and gnawing. It occurs mostly during bedtime, but it can also happen when you are busy with something else. Some experience it while watching TV or sitting in a car.
- **Urge to move:** In order to relieve the discomfort; you'll feel the urge to constantly move your legs or arms. This urge often feels uncontrollable, and it increases when lying down or sitting still. Trying not to move tends to only worsen the symptoms.
- **Sleepiness:** Since it greatly affects the quality of your sleep, you will experience a lot of daytime sleepiness, and you might require naps to make it through the day. You might also experience severe drowsiness and tend to yawn in conversations with others.
- **Performance problems:** It's really hard to stay concentrated when you're tired or when you experience restless legs syndrome. That's why many people who suffer from restless legs syndrome have work performance issues and

might even experience behavioral issues due to exhaustion.

- **Bedtime issues:** When you suffer from restless legs syndrome, you'll often find yourself uncomfortable when you start to get tired. That means you might get up a couple of times to walk around, stretch, or even do another activity to distract your mind from the discomfort and soothe the pain. Naturally, this affects the quality of your sleep and can cause some bedtime issues.

- **Sleep disruption:** In some cases, restless legs syndrome can keep you awake or even wake you up once you've fallen asleep. Constant sleep disruption can lead to exhaustion and other severe sleep disorders. Since you are also more likely to get out of bed a couple of times in order to soothe discomfort, you will spend less time actually resting.

- **Changes in mood:** Restless legs syndrome can greatly influence your moods, and it can lead to depression and anxiety. Due to a loss of sleep, you might often find yourself exhausted, unmotivated, and in a dark space. You'll start losing interest in the things that you enjoy due to being scared of struggling with your legs.

SICK AND TIRED | 65

Now that we've looked at the most common sleep disorders, it's time to look at why they really matter. Researchers believe that sleep disorders aren't just uncomfortable and lead to exhaustion and being sleep-deprived; they can actually lead to other illnesses. In the next section, we'll look at the connection between these sleep disorders we just discussed and other illnesses.

CONNECTION BETWEEN SLEEP DISORDERS AND OTHER ILLNESSES

There's a reason we feel grumpy after a night of very little sleep but imagine going for weeks or even months without proper sleep! What would the effects be? Well, since you're here, you probably have a pretty clear picture of how it might feel to suffer from inconsistent sleep over a long period of time. I remember feeling so tired that it was hard even to spend time with my family. I could never stay awake during a family movie and would often disappear to the bedroom as soon as I had the chance to get some sleep. Well, it turns out that many other illnesses are actually connected to a lack of sleep and experiencing sleep disorders.

Specifically, there are four illnesses most commonly caused by a sleep disorder:

- depression

- anxiety
- heart disease
- diabetes

Sleep and Depression

Depression can be identified as persistent sadness, disappointment, and hopelessness. It affects you emotionally, mentally, and physically, and it can lead to isolation. Depression can also lead to life-threatening behavior and is classified as a mood disorder (Newsom, 2020). Depression and sleep troubles often go hand in hand. In many cases, people with depression find it hard to sleep at night and experience extreme daytime struggles. The other side of the coin is that sleep struggles can also lead to depression. The two create a cycle that influences each other constantly. According to the Sleep Foundation, depression, and sleep are closely connected, and a majority of people with depression also experience sleeping disorders. Just like in the case of the chicken and the egg, it's hard to determine which one was first.

Depression is most commonly associated with insomnia and obstructive sleep apnea. Almost 20% of people with depression have sleep apnea, which influences the brain and neurotransmitters. The less quality sleep you get, the more vulnerable you are to depression. On top of that, almost 80% of people with depression struggle with insomnia (Newsom, 2020). Since one influences the other, it's essential to find a way to stop the cycle. Once the cycle is stopped, the symptoms will lessen, and treatment can take place.

Sleep and Anxiety

Anxiety and sleeping problems are closely connected and often seen together in patients. When you have anxiety, you have an excess of worry and fear, which makes it harder to fall asleep and stay asleep. When you have anxiety, sleep deprivation can worsen, which spurs the negative cycle of anxiety and insomnia (Suni, 2020). Anxiety is a prevalent mental disorder globally, and it has a lot of negative health implications. Insomnia is considered a common symptom of anxiety, and people often lay in bed at night, unable to switch off their minds. When your mind is hyperarousal, you will have high sleep reactivity, meaning you will sleep very lightly and wake up feeling panicked. When stress increases, anxiety worsens, which in turn also worsens insomnia. When you know you struggle to fall asleep, you might start to avoid going to bed or trying to sleep due to the anxiety it gives you.

Anxiety also influences your REM sleep and causes you to experience more vivid dreams and nightmares. You might find yourself waking up multiple times a night after experiencing a vivid dream or feeling like you just thought yourself awake (Suni, 2020). Insomnia worsens the anxiety symptoms and once again creates a negative cycle where the two disorders greatly influence each other. Sleep apnea can also lead to anxiety because you are scared that you might stop breathing and die.

Sleep and Heart Disease

Not getting adequate sleep can lead to serious heart disease. Good sleep isn't just essential for day-to-day functioning; it can also help your heart stay healthy. In many cases, heart disease starts with unhealthy sleeping patterns and bad sleep hygiene. Staying up later to watch a movie or not prioritizing rest places your heart under a lot of pressure. Poor sleep can even lead to higher rates of arrhythmia, pulmonary hypertension, and atrial fibrillation (Lui, 2022). When you don't sleep enough, you will experience more inflammation in your body, which can cause high blood pressure. High blood pressure also comes with the risk of heart failure and heart disease.

When you treat your sleep disorder as a serious issue, you will be able to regulate your blood pressure and aid in the health of your heart. However, if you fail to recognize its importance, you might end up neglecting your sleep habits even more and placing your heart under more pressure. There are many healthy habits that you can implement to increase both your heart health and your sleep patterns. These habits include exercising, prioritizing a healthy diet, and quitting smoking. The first step is to make sure you get into bed by 10 p.m.

Sleep and Diabetes

Diabetes affects millions of people, and it is the seventh leading cause of death in the United States. Type 2 diabetes is the most common form of diabetes, and it develops due to insulin resistance. Insulin is the hormone that transfers glucose from the blood to the muscles. It helps your body get the energy that it needs to do its tasks (Pacheco, 2022). Many people with type 2 diabetes also experience insomnia and other sleeping disorders. The reason for this is due to blood sugar levels being unstable, which causes an irregular pattern of sleep. When your blood sugar is high, your kidneys need to overcompensate and create more urine. This causes you to run to the bathroom multiple times a night, interrupting your sleep. It can also cause headaches and fatigue.

Low blood sugar, on the other hand, can cause nightmares, sweating, and feelings of confusion, all of which can wake you up at night and interrupt your sleep. When you don't get proper sleep, it negatively impacts your blood sugar levels, and it can cause high blood sugar levels. As you can see, once again, the two elements influence each other negatively. Poor sleep also increases the risk of obesity, which is another risk factor for diabetes.

As you can see, getting enough sleep isn't just a nice idea; it can save your life. The sleeping disorders we discussed in this chapter can influence the way our body works and can cause many health risks in our lives. That's why it's so essential to define the sleeping disorder that we're struggling with and take the appropriate steps to improve our health and our sleep patterns. Luckily, we can do something about that. In the next chapter, we'll look at five lifestyle changes that can transform the way we sleep for the better. No matter what sleeping disorder you might be experiencing, these five lifestyle changes will be able to help you get on the right track. Are you ready to transform your lifestyle into one that welcomes sleep? Let's do it!

3

THE 5 LIFESTYLE CHANGES FOR BETTER SLEEP

Habits are formed by the repetition of particular acts. They are strengthened by an increase in the number of repeated acts. Habits are also weakened or broken, and contrary habits are formed by the repetition of contrary acts.

— MORTIMER J. ADLER

I f you want to change your sleep patterns, you need to start by addressing your sleep habits. We all build sleep habits, regardless of whether we're trying to or not. The only difference is the intention behind the habits. If we allow natural habits to form, they'll most likely not be super healthy or beneficial to our sleep health. However, when we focus on building habits that contribute to better sleep, it's worth giving it a try, don't you think?

Years ago, I visited an old friend of mine who lived across the country. We decided to finally catch up while I was on a work break, and he invited me to stay with him for the weekend. It was glorious seeing him again and catching up on the past years, and the first night I spent with him and his family, we stayed up and talked until well after midnight. I knew I was in for a long night when he made us strong coffee around 10 p.m. The next evening, I was utterly knackered and exhausted. I excused myself right after 10 p.m. and slept like a baby (with my mask). Somewhere in the early hours of the morning, I woke up with a thirst that needed to be quenched immediately. I walked to the kitchen to get some water, and to my surprise, I found my friend on the couch in front of the TV, still in his clothes from the previous evening. It turns out he never goes to bed before 2 a.m. and prefers falling asleep on the couch with the TV on.

Two days later, he confided in me and shared with me how he was struggling with his health. "I'm always sick and irritated," he said. He claimed that he had no idea why he felt this way or why he was even starting to feel isolated and depressed. As gently as I could, I told him that was probably because of his sleep hygiene. He laughed it off and said that it couldn't be that since he naturally adopted his sleep routine. Well, skip forward a couple of months, and you'll find my friend in a hospital bed calling me to tell me that I was right. It was his sleep habits all along.

Our sleeping habits shouldn't be misjudged or taken for granted just because they happen naturally or are formulated on their own. What worked for you in your teenage years might not work for your body anymore, so you need to adjust your habits. That's what this chapter is all about. We'll discuss the five lifestyle changes that you need to apply to your daily life in order to improve your sleep. The five lifestyle changes we'll look at include

- establishing sleep hygiene
- the role of exercise
- the importance of your diet
- the role of nutrient supplementation
- the benefits of relaxing

LIFESTYLE CHANGE 1: THE POWER OF SLEEP HYGIENE

Sleep hygiene is the first step you should take when working toward better sleep. Sleep hygiene means creating a bedroom environment and a daily routine that promotes consistent, uninterrupted sleep (Suni, 2020a). When you think of the word "hygiene," it usually refers to cleanliness and keeping yourself fresh. Well, in the case of sleep hygiene, the goal is to keep your sleep "clean" by setting up your sleep for success. Certain habits and routines can either contribute to better sleep or hinder it. For example, if you have an espresso at 10 p.m.—that's not very sleep-hygienic of you.

Sleep hygiene is essential for physical and mental health. It also improves productivity and quality of life (Suni, 2020a). Sleep hygiene is one of the best ways to work toward better sleep, even if you suffer from a sleeping disorder. You might look at your current sleep habits and realize that your sleep hygiene isn't great. Well, luckily, we have the ability to change those habits. By being intentional and working toward better sleep, we can implement certain habits that will help us achieve our sleep goals.

If you're not sure whether your sleep hygiene is good or bad, here are a couple of signs that you might not have great sleep hygiene (Suni, 2020a).

- You have a hard time falling asleep.
- You experience frequent sleep disruptions and disturbances.
- You find it hard to stay awake during the day.
- Feeling tired when waking up.
- Having no consistency in your sleep.

So, what can we do to implement this lifestyle change of good sleep hygiene? Well, there are a couple of ways that we can improve our sleep, and it all starts with building consistency. Let's have a look at six ways that you can incorporate better sleep hygiene today.

Start a Schedule

The first step to good sleep hygiene is to incorporate a sleep schedule. A sleep schedule is a guide that tells you when to go to bed and when to wake up. The goal is to build consistency and help your body get used to the sleep schedule. Keeping a regular sleep schedule can be pretty tricky, especially when the weekend rolls in, but it's essential if you want to maintain good sleep hygiene. When you sleep on a schedule, your body will start to adjust and send the right hormones at the right time to aid you in your sleep. By being consistent, your body will be less likely to fight you to stay awake at night, especially if you wake up at the same time. Instead of sleeping in on the weekend, get up at your regular times to improve your sleep drive for the next night (Headspace, 2023).

Pre-bedtime Routine

A bedtime routine might sound silly, but many experts believe that having an excellent bedtime routine can significantly decrease your chances of struggling with sleeping disorders. Keeping your routine consistent is especially important. A routine is basically how you prepare yourself for bed. Do you watch TV until you pass out? Or do you follow a routine to make sure that your mind and body are relaxed and ready to rest? A good bedtime routine consists of a shower or bath and putting on clothes dedicated to sleeping (don't just sleep in your shirt and sweatpants). It's also important to say goodbye to all screens at least 30 minutes before you get into bed. A good bedtime routine can also make use of relaxation methods like reading or guided meditation. Your bedtime routine is a way for you to signal your body and your brain that it's time to switch off and get into bed. That's why it's essential that you stick to your routine and be consistent with its implementation (Stibich, 2021).

Invest in Your Environment

Your bedroom shouldn't be the storage space for everything that doesn't have a place somewhere else. In fact, your bedroom should be an oasis where you can relax, not be reminded of the things you didn't do. Your bedroom should represent tranquility and peace, so invest in it. Make sure that it looks appealing and creates a safe space for you to relax. Don't put the exercise bike in there! That will only make you feel guilty for not using it for years. Instead, make sure that your room is clean and comfortable. Think about it; you spend a third of your life in bed! So, why not invest in a bed that's comfortable? Make sure that the linen on your bed is enjoyable and not irritating to your skin. Investing in your bedroom is a great way to make sure that you prioritize sleep. When you step into your bedroom, you should sense immediate relaxation and calmness. What can you do to make your bedroom more inviting today?

Dim the Lights

A great way to ensure sleep hygiene is by dimming your bedroom lights. While you're winding down, turn off those harsh lights and turn on a softer, more relaxing light. By dimming the lights, your body will create more hormones to help you fall asleep (Suni, 2020a). Bright lights prevent this hormone from being released, so be sure to dim those lights as soon as you get into the room. A dimmed light will also help you relax, so put away those harsh screen lights and enjoy the soft glow of the bedside lamp.

Unplug

Speaking of lights and devices, it's essential that you unplug at least 30 minutes before bedtime. If you can, implement a device-free rule in your bedroom where you don't take your phone or laptop into your bedroom. Your screens cause mental stimulation, which ultimately keeps you awake. So, when you're on your phone right before bed, your brain will have difficulty shutting off. Instead of scrolling on your phone before bed, try to do something else instead, like reading or journaling. When you use a device, the blue light interferes with the release of melatonin, which is the hormone that makes you sleepy. According to Dr. Ronal Chervin, you should aim to be screen-free for at least 45 minutes prior to bedtime (Kaufman, 2023). So, if you're using your phone as your alarm clock and scrolling endlessly at night, invest in an old-school alarm and leave your phone by the door.

Limit Your Naps

Naps can be greatly beneficial, and they can especially help you get through the day when you're experiencing extreme exhaustion. However, it's important to limit your naps and not sleep for more than 20 to 30 minutes. Try to avoid taking longer naps that might cause you to not be tired by bedtime. A 20-minute nap will replenish enough energy for you to make it through the rest of the day without damaging your nightly sleep. Try to limit your naps to the earlier side of the day and avoid having a nap after 3 p.m.

With these simple practices, you can begin to improve your sleep hygiene and experience better sleep patterns. Now that we've covered the first lifestyle change that you need to make in order to experience better sleep, it's time to look at lifestyle change two.

LIFESTYLE CHANGE 2: THE ROLE OF EXERCISE

I know no one wants to hear it, but exercise is actually essential and healthy for us. Look, I like running around and sweating like a racehorse as much as the next guy, but when you experience how good exercise is for your sleep, things begin to change. Exercise can alleviate sleep-related problems, and it can even help you get an adequate amount of sleep at night (Pacheco, 2021). Sleep and exercise have a bidirectional relationship, meaning that they influence each other significantly. When you're tired, you don't want to exercise, and when you don't exercise, you don't sleep as well at night. It's a nasty cycle that needs to be interrupted at some point. Moderate exercise can increase the quality of sleep for many people, and it can even decrease the amount of time that you lie awake at night. Exercise can also help alleviate daytime drowsiness and, in some cases, reduce the need for medication. Exercise can also decrease stress in your life, which also contributes to a better quality of sleep (Pacheco, 2021). However, when is the best time to exercise, and how much exercise do we need? Luckily for you, I have the answers right here!

When to Exercise?

The answer to this question is simple: any exercise is better than no exercise, so find a time slot that works for you. Many people believe that exercising late at night can be harmful to their sleep, while others believe that it contributes to better sleep. The truth is, it might differ from person to person, so the best time to exercise is when you most enjoy doing so. If your schedule is jam-packed and you only have time to exercise in the morning, then you do that. But if you prefer exercising after work or even after dinner, that's okay too. Whatever works for you is excellent! In general, exercising will contribute to better sleep, regardless of when you exercise as long as you leave yourself enough time to cool down and bring your heart rate back to normal before you get in bed. When you exercise right before bedtime, your temperature might be quite high, which can lead to less deep sleep. So, to recap, exercise whenever you can, but allow yourself enough time to cool down before getting into your bedtime routine (Pacheco, 2021).

How Much Should I Exercise?

Depending on the type of exercise, how much exercise you need might vary. However, the Centers for Disease Control and Prevention suggest that adults get at least 3 hours of exercise a week. However, even working out for 10 minutes a day can be beneficial to your health (Okoye, 2017). Doing one single exercise might influence your sleep for one night, but having a continuous routine of exercising will be more beneficial to your health. Exercises that improve sleep include the following (Okoye, 2017):

- **Cardio:** Any exercise that focuses on increasing your heart rate is considered cardio. That includes walking, running, swimming, and team sports like basketball and soccer. Long-term cardio can improve your sleep and promote healthier sleep hygiene.
- **Resistance Training:** Resistance training involves muscle-strengthening exercises and is

known for improving your quality of sleep. Resistance training includes weight training and using resistance bands. If you enjoy gardening, a good day's work also counts as resistance training!

- **Mind-Body Exercise:** Exercises that include the mind are known to improve sleep and can help people who suffer from insomnia. Exercises include yoga, tai chi, and qigong.

By implementing this lifestyle change, you'll start to experience better sleep and improved sleep hygiene.

LIFESTYLE CHANGE 3: THE IMPORTANCE OF YOUR DIET

Nutrition plays a fundamental role in your health, even though its importance is often overlooked. Your diet can influence the quality of your sleep, and some foods and drinks can even prevent it. It's essential that we recognize the connection between sleep and nutrition, which starts by understanding what nutrition really is. There are three parts to nutrition that we need to grasp (Suni, 2020b):

- **Macronutrients:** Macronutrients include carbohydrates, protein, and amino acids.

- **Vitamins:** Vitamins play a very important role in our bodies, and there are 13 essential vitamins that we need to receive on a daily basis.
- **Minerals:** Minerals are needed to power different systems in the body, and they can be classified as macrominerals.

What you eat on a daily basis serves as the backbone of your health. What you eat will either result in you having enough energy or your body not functioning properly. Your diet greatly affects your sleep since it can either contribute to better sleep or disrupt it. Let's have a closer look at which foods help you sleep and which foods you should probably avoid if you want to sleep better.

Foods That Help You Sleep

The best way to ensure healthy sleep through nutrition is by eating a balanced diet. One of the best diets to ensure balance is the Mediterranean diet, which is filled with plant-based foods and healthy fats. People who stick to the Mediterranean diet are less likely to suffer from a sleeping disorder. More specifically, there are different kinds of foods that can aid in the quality of your sleep:

- **Tryptophan:** Your tryptophan levels influence your sleep, so it's important to eat food with high tryptophan levels. This includes foods like meat, seeds, nuts, eggs, and cheese.
- **Fruits and Vegetables:** Everyone knows that fruits and vegetables are essential when you're trying to maintain a balanced diet, but eating fruit and vegetables can also improve your sleep. When you don't get a lot of fruit and vegetables, you are more likely to suffer from sleep disorders.
- **Kiwi:** Kiwi fruits offer a lot of health benefits. Eating a Kiwi before bed can provide sleep benefits such as sleeping longer and falling asleep faster.
- **Cherries:** Cherries contain high levels of melatonin and serotonin, which play a significant role in better sleep. When you eat cherries, your sleep quality will improve instantly. Other foods with high levels of melatonin include grapes, strawberries, tomatoes, and peppers.
- **Fish:** Oily fish such as sardines and salmon can also help you sleep better, especially if you're older than 40.
- **Herbal teas:** Certain teas are known to help with sleeping disorders. Chamomile tea has

great benefits, and it also helps you fall asleep easier. Other teas are also great to drink in the afternoon since they don't contain caffeine.

- **Carbohydrates:** Research has found that insomnia is less common among people who eat more whole grains. However, some carbs can increase sleeplessness, so try to avoid sugar and refined grains.

By prioritizing these foods and adding them to your daily diet, you're one step closer to experiencing better-quality sleep. Next, let's look at the foods you should avoid.

Food That Disrupts Your Sleep

Some foods can greatly disrupt your sleep and your sleeping patterns. Some of these are pretty well known, but some of these foods are quite surprising and have a way of sneaking into our meals:

- **Fatty foods:** The first thing we need to avoid are fatty foods. Consuming a lot of saturated and trans fats can lead to reduced sleep times and sleeping disorders. Fatty foods are mostly animal products, like cheese, meat, and fried food.

- **Alcohol:** The next food that you need to avoid in order to improve your sleep is alcohol. While winding down the day with a glass of wine might sound fantastic, it can greatly affect your sleep in a negative way. Oftentimes, alcohol makes us feel drowsy, but as soon as the effects wear off, you'll find yourself waking up and struggling with restless sleep. Alcohol can also increase your sleeping disorder.
- **Caffeine:** This culprit is one most of us are aware of. Drinking caffeine late in the day can be a great sleep disruptor, stimulate your brain, and keep you awake. Caffeine is often hidden in other foods, like chocolate and ice cream, so be careful what you eat late at night. Caffeine isn't only in coffee and energy drinks, so take a close look at your ingredients before indulging.
- **Spicy food:** For some people, spicy food can cause heartburn, which makes it uncomfortable to lie down and fall asleep. Heartburn can also increase the symptoms of sleep apnea, which can also disrupt your sleep. On top of that, spicy food will raise your temperature and force your body to work harder to keep you cool. This extra stress on your body can lead to disrupted sleep patterns throughout the night.

- **Processed food:** The last food you want to avoid in order to improve your sleep is food that is heavily processed. Processed food contains a lot of sugar and other ingredients that act as preservatives but also keep you awake. It's also harder for your body to process already processed foods, which takes an extra toll on what your body is doing while you're sleeping. Processed food might cause indigestion, which will also affect the quality of your sleep.

By avoiding these foods and making sure you eat enough of the foods that promote sleep, you'll be able to take better care of your sleep habits and improve your overall quality of sleep.

LIFESTYLE CHANGE 4: THE ROLE OF NUTRIENT SUPPLEMENTATION

Supplementation isn't the same as just food; that's why it requires a whole lifestyle change on its own. Some supplements that we take might be keeping us awake without us even noticing it. Other supplements can actually aid in our sleep. We just need to know which supplements to look for and which ones to avoid. Even though the best way to consume nutrients is through the meals that you're eating, nutritional supplements can help you reach better sleep quality sooner. Some supplements to help with sleep include

- melatonin
- magnesium
- valerian root
- glycine
- tryptophan
- ginkgo biloba
- lavender
- passionflower

Before adding any supplement to your diet, be sure to check with your doctor to see whether they would recommend it and what they would recommend. Remember, our bodies work differently and might respond differently to certain supplements. It's best to check in with your doctor and confirm with them before adding any supplements to your diet.

LIFESTYLE CHANGE 5: THE BENEFITS OF RELAXING

The final lifestyle change that you need to make in order to improve your sleep is to understand and implement relaxation techniques. When you're able to truly relax, you will experience loads of benefits, all of which contribute to the quality of your sleep. Some benefits of relaxation techniques include (Mayo Clinic, 2017):

- lower blood pressure
- boost in confidence
- slowing breathing rate
- slowing heart rate
- improving digestion
- better blood sugar levels and balance
- reducing muscle tension and chronic pain
- reducing stress hormones
- improving mood
- improving sleep quality and reducing fatigue

There are different types of relaxation methods and techniques that you can incorporate into your daily life. Let's have a closer look at a couple of relaxation methods, according to the Mayo Clinic (2017).

Autogenic Relaxation

The word autogenic means that it's something that comes from within you. In other words, this relaxation method focuses on what comes from inside you and how you are aware of your body. Autogenic relaxation involves repeating certain calming words over and over again to yourself until you feel your body respond accordingly. Close your eyes, imagine a peaceful setting, and repeat calming words to yourself. Then, take note of your heart rate slowing down, your tension releasing, and your muscles relaxing (Mayo Clinic, 2017). Repeat the calming words over and over again until you feel relaxed.

Progressive Muscle Relaxation

This relaxation technique requires you to focus on tensing and releasing your muscles. You'll focus on one muscle group at a time. Start with your feet as you flex, then relax them. Become aware of your muscles and how they're feeling, and be sure to end in a relaxing state. Progressively work your way up until you reach the top of your head. Focus on tensing the muscles in your neck and then releasing them (Mayo Clinic, 2017). Allow the feeling of relaxation to flow through your whole body as you embrace peace and calm. This relaxation method is wonderful after a rough day since you can do it wherever you are.

Visualization

Visualization is all about forming pictures in your mind and seeing a picture that is peaceful, calming, and relaxing. You can use your senses to help you visualize. For example, let's say you're visualizing the beach. What do you see? Focus on the waves and the bright sun. Perhaps you're spotting some dolphins in the waves. Then focus on the sound. Listen to the waves as they crash onto the beach. Focus on hearing the seagulls as they fly around. What do you feel? Visualize the feeling of the sand underneath you and the hot sun warming you up. Next, what do you smell? Visualize the fresh smell of the ocean and the sweet smell of the ice cream in your hand. Finally, what do you taste? Perhaps the salty water on your lips or the ice cream you're enjoying.

Visualization is a powerful tool that can help you focus on the positive and remain calm, despite what you're facing. It's also a great way to turn away from the struggles and distractions of the day and just calm your mind.

Breathing Exercises

Taking a deep breath is so underrated! If we fully understood the power of deep breathing, we'd all make it mandatory to practice breathing at least once a day. Breathing exercises can calm you down, help you focus, and even remove anxiety. I have a friend who has struggled with horrible nightmares ever since she was a little girl. When she wakes up at night due to a terrible nightmare, she jumps up, turns on the lights, and tries to distract herself from the fear she's feeling. As you can imagine, the bright lights and sudden fight-or-flight actions usually lead to her not being able to fall asleep again. A couple of years ago, she decided to do deep breathing exercises before she went to bed and to take ten deep breaths after waking up from a nightmare before putting on the lights. As it turns out, after ten deep breaths, she was able to control her fear, calm her mind, and focus on reality. After a couple of minutes, she would peacefully fall back asleep.

You can also incorporate breathing exercises, regardless of where you are or what you're doing. One of my favorite things to do is practice deep breathing as I'm driving to and from work. This puts me in a space of calm and not panic before I enter the work environment, and on the way home, it helps me to leave work at the office and not bring it with me mentally. My favorite breathing exercise is square breathing. Imagine drawing a square in your mind. As you draw the first vertical line, breathe in for 4 seconds. As you draw your first horizontal line, hold your breath for 4 seconds. As you exhale for 4 seconds, you're drawing the second vertical line, going down. Finally, keep your lungs empty for four seconds. Then repeat the square a couple of times. This breathing exercise is a great way to take control of your anxious and racing mind and focus on relaxing.

Meditation

The final relaxation method I would suggest is meditation. While many of us might be hesitant to try meditating due to not being 100% comfortable with it or not knowing what to expect, meditation is a wonderful way to relax. There are so many different types of meditation that can be beneficial for you. You can make use of guided meditations by downloading an app like Balance or Headspace. You can also meditate on your own by finding a quiet place, closing your eyes, and focusing on letting go of everything. Yoga and mindfulness exercises are also part of meditating, so you don't have to do anything you're not comfortable with. If you're spiritual and religious, you can also use meditation as part of your religious practices.

There you have it: The five lifestyle changes that can improve the quality of your sleep in no time. These lifestyle changes might not be the cure for any sleeping disorder that you might be experiencing, but they can help with the symptoms and make them more bearable. Besides, what if it helps? What if these simple changes would change your sleep forever? Isn't it worth finding that out? Of course it is! So, don't wait until you are so tired you can barely function. Rather, start by incorporating these lifestyle changes one at a time. In the next chapter, we'll look at possible medications that can help with sleeping disorders, but first, it's time for a quick interactive element.

MY CHANGE STARTS TODAY

I want to encourage you to choose one of these five lifestyle changes and dedicate yourself to applying that change this week. You don't have to implement all of these changes at once, but it's important that we start somewhere. Write down which lifestyle you want to change, and then create a short list with actionable things that you should aim for this week. Keep track of how it influences your sleep and whether you can feel a difference.

4

MEDICATION FOR SLEEP DISORDERS

There's a heartwarming story of a woman named Suzanne Reagan, who was nicknamed "Sleeping Beauty" by her friends and teachers. Suzanne often fell asleep in class, despite her best attempts to stay awake. Her older sister suffered from the same thing. In fact, she was used to recording all her classes to make sure that she never missed anything important. Upon closer inspection, Suzanne started realizing that her mom also napped almost every day and would always fall asleep during a movie. A couple of years went by before Suzanne's older sister was diagnosed with narcolepsy. Suzanne immediately knew she had to be tested as well and got her diagnosis soon after. Working closely with her healthcare providers, Suzanne was prescribed medication that helped her sleep at night and stay awake during the day. Suzanne confirmed that even though most medications have side effects, she'd be forever grateful for the medication since she can now live her life like a normal person and take part in daily activities without being scared that she might fall asleep (Cleveland Clinic, 2023).

As we can see in Suzanne's case, medication helped her treat her sleeping disorder and continue with her life. I can also testify to how medications helped me with my sleeping disorders. In this chapter, we'll discuss the pros and cons of medication. We'll also look at over-the-counter medication as well as prescription medication and how it can help with your sleep quality. My goal is not to convince you to use medication but rather to be transparent with you and give you all the options necessary to make this decision. Let's start by looking at over-the-counter medication and its effect on people with sleep disorders.

OVER-THE-COUNTER MEDICATION

If you've been struggling with your sleep disorder for a while, you might have already checked out over-the-counter (OTC) medication. However, it can be scary to try to medicate. Questions like, "Is it safe?" or "Will it really work?" tend to circle the drain, and we find ourselves even more overwhelmed and confused. Well, allow me to shed some light on the matter. Most medications that you can buy over-the-counter for sleep are considered safe. However, each medication comes with its own risks and side effects. The most common side effect of OTC medication is daytime grogginess. For some people, it can even cause confusion and blurred vision. Besides the side effects (which we'll talk about more later), OTC medication is usually not very helpful with long-term chronic sleep disorders. If you've had a bad night or two, it can work wonders. However, it might be best to seek a better long-term solution. Let's have a closer look at the most common OTC medications and the risks they might contain.

Most Common

There are dozens of OCT medications to choose from to aid in falling asleep. However, they can all be classified into one of the following categories:

- **Melatonin:** Melatonin might sound familiar to you, and that's because we spoke about it earlier on this journey. Melatonin is a natural hormone that is usually produced in the pineal gland of the brain. When we're awake, our retinas perceive light as a sign to be awake and

then create other hormones to balance out the
melatonin production that happens during the
night. However, there are many factors that can
influence the production of melatonin. Things
like being exposed to a bright light might leave
your brain thinking it's daytime, releasing the
wrong hormone. Melatonin in medication can
help you balance your sleep better, and it's
especially great when people are jet-lagged.
However, melatonin is a blood-thinning agent,
so if you suffer from epilepsy or are on other
blood-thinning medications, this might not be
the best option for you (Pacheco, 2020).

- **Diphenhydramine:** The next category of OTC
  medications is diphenhydramine, which is an
  FDA-approved antihistamine. The most
  common brand of diphenhydramine is
  Benadryl. It can also be found in many pain-
  relieving or fever-reducing medications.
  However, the effectiveness of diphenhydramine
  on sleep is debatable. While some people would
  sleep peacefully after taking it, others wouldn't
  feel affected at all. When taken over a long
  period of time, it can be problematic. As we get
  older, our metabolisms slowdown, which
  means that the drowsiness might only appear
  later, causing you to be sleepy during the day.

SICK AND TIRED | 99

When taken too often, diphenhydramine can lead to heart problems, going into a coma, and experiencing a seizure (Pacheco, 2020).

- **Doxylamine:** Doxylamine is also a first-generation antihistamine that produces sedative effects. Doxylamine can work as a short-term treatment for insomnia and can also be used to alleviate cold symptoms. However, doxylamine isn't recommended for use for more than two weeks at a time. If taken over a longer period, it can lead to problematic heart conditions. Some of the most well-known brands of doxylamine are Unisom, Medi-Sleep, and Good Sense Sleep Aid (Pacheco, 2020).

- **Valerian:** Next on the list is Valerian, which is a dietary supplement. Best known as valerian root, it is often used to treat anxiety or insomnia. Valerian interacts with your brain's receptors, which helps it reduce cortisol, the stress hormone. Since valerian root is a supplement and not a medication, it has not been evaluated by the FDA as a sleeping aid. When you take too much valerian, it can lead to morning drowsiness, but if you use the correct amount, you'll feel alert and more focused in the morning. The effects of valerian have not yet been tested on children or pregnant women, so it's best to stay clear of valerian if you are expecting or breastfeeding (Pacheco, 2020).

- **Chamomile:** This flower has been used for thousands of years to help people relax and increase sleep quality. It can also be taken in pill form, but the most popular use of chamomile is in tea. Many people with sleep problems might drink some chamomile before bed in the hopes that it will improve their sleep. Chamomile is relatively safe, although some people might have an allergic reaction to the flower.

- **CBD:** Derivative of the cannabis plant, can now be found as an over-the-counter medication and in other health shops. CBD does not include the THC of the plant, which is the ingredient that causes the "high." CBD can be used in the form of a pill, a drink, a cream, or edible sweets like gummies. CBD can also help relieve anxiety, which is a big contributor to sleep quality. For some people, CBD is still a very scary thought since they connect it with illegal drugs and smoking marijuana. However, if you have no moral objections and want to try something natural, CBD is a great avenue to explore first. CBD can be quite expensive, though (Shaw, 2018).

Risks

Like most medications, over-the-counter sleep aids can have side effects and risks. The tricky thing with side effects and risks is that different people respond completely differently to the same medication. Some common side effects of over-the-counter sleep aids are dry mouth, urinary retention, constipation, and blurred vision (Boland, 2021). Here are a couple of potential side effects of some of the most popular over-the-counter sleep aid categories, as we described in the previous section (Shaw, 2018):

- Melatonin can cause feelings of depression, dizziness, daytime sleepiness, headaches, and nausea. In some cases, it can also lead to enuresis, which is adult bedwetting.
- Diphenhydramine can also lead to dizziness, coordination problems, epigastric pain, and a thickening of bronchial secretions.
- Doxylamine can lead to drowsiness and dizziness as well, but it also includes the possibility of thickening of mucus in the nose and throat, as well as dry mouth, throat, and nose.
- Valerian root can lead to an upset stomach, confusion, a strange sense of excitement, strange dreams, and headaches.

- Chamomile can lead to nausea and an allergic reaction in some people. In some cases, it can also cause dizziness.
- CBD can cause diarrhea, reduced appetite, fatigue, drowsiness, and dry mouth.

Precautions to Keep in Mind

When you're ready to try an over-the-counter medication to aid in your sleep, there are a couple of things that you should keep in mind. See these guidelines as precautions to ensure your own safety and health. At the end of the day, medication isn't something to play around with; it's something to be taken seriously and respected. Let's take a look at a couple of precautions as suggested by the Mayo Clinic (2019):

- Start by having a conversation with your healthcare provider. Make sure that your sleep aid won't interact negatively with some of the other medications you might be taking for underlying conditions by being transparent with your healthcare provider. You can also ask them for advice on dosage and which type of sleep aid they would recommend.
- The second precaution to keep in mind is to make sure you are aware of possible side effects and that you know how the specific aid you'll

be using might affect your health. Some aids aren't suited for people with other underlying problems, like low blood pressure. Do your research, and be sure to check out recommendations from experts. This is especially important if you're older than 65.

- Take it one day at a time, and don't expect to be magically saved from sleep deprivation after one night of using a sleeping aid. Allow it time to work, and don't jump between different aids all the time. Nonprescription sleep aids aren't meant to be used long-term, so if it goes beyond a temporary solution, I suggest getting a script for something else.

- Lastly, it's essential that you don't mix sleep aids with alcohol. Alcohol can greatly increase the sedative effect and lead to some serious dangers, so rather stay away completely.

When you don't find a temporary solution, it might be time to see your doctor and get some prescription medication. However, if you're willing to try the OTC medications first, give them a try! Perhaps some chamomile tea is all your body needs. Next, we'll look at prescription medication.

PRESCRIPTION MEDICATION

Prescription medication is only available at pharmacies, and you need an order from a doctor for a specific medication in order to receive that medication. Prescription medication is closely monitored by the FDA, which gives it a little bit more safety and security than other possibilities. There are many prescription drugs to aid in sleep quality, each with its own pros and cons. Prescription medication alters your brain chemicals, which then aid in your sleep. Let's have a look at a couple of types of prescription medication that can be used for sleep problems.

Most Common

Depending on your healthcare provider and your specific sleep disorder, you'll be prescribed a different type of medication. However, there are a few different types that you can be aware of and prepare yourself for in order to know exactly what you're getting yourself into and what you should expect. Educating yourself on the different types of prescription medication can help you understand the whole journey a little bit better. There are six categories that prescription sleep medication can fall into:

- **Hypnotics and Sedatives:** The first type of prescription medication is hypnotics and sedatives, which are drugs that are designed to make you feel sleepy (Suni, 2020c). Benzodiazepines are considered the first generation of hypnotics and sedatives, and they work by increasing your brain's production of gamma-aminobutyric acid, which is the chemical in your body that induces drowsiness. However, in recent years, new hypnotics have been discovered and are more commonly prescribed since they have fewer side effects than benzodiazepines. Hypnotic drugs are fast acting, but some are created to be slow-releasing, depending on whether you have trouble staying asleep or falling asleep (Suni, 2020c). There are other sedatives that are more effective in making people fall asleep, but they're not the first choice of treatment since they can be highly addictive.
- **Orexin Receptor Antagonist:** The second type of hypnotics and sedatives are orexin receptor antagonists. Orexin is a natural substance that increases wakefulness, so this drug works as an antagonist by blocking the effect of orexin. This type of drug decreases the levels of orexin in the body, which promotes sleep without some

of the side effects that might occur with other sleeping agents. Orexin receptor antagonists are less likely to cause headaches, nausea, and short-term forgetfulness than hypnotics (Suni, 2020c). However, if your sleeping disorder is severe, this drug alone might not work best for you.

- **Melatonin Receptor Agonist:** Melatonin is a naturally produced hormone in the body that works almost as the opposite of orexin. Melatonin facilitates the body's ability to sleep and maintain a steady circadian rhythm (Suni, 2020c). In other words, a melatonin receptor agonist mimics the effect of the melatonin in your body, causing you to fall asleep and be drowsy. This is mostly used for people who struggle with falling asleep. Even though you can get melatonin over the counter, the prescription drug is much more effective and different than the melatonin supplement.
- **Antidepressant:** Even though antidepressants are created and developed to treat depression, most antidepressants include a sedative that can cause drowsiness in some people. Therefore, antidepressants are often prescribed for sleeping problems and to address other sleeping issues. Antidepressants have not yet been

approved by the FDA as sleeping agents, which means that this is an "off the label" use of the product. When you use a product "off the label," you take it to treat something that it wasn't technically created for. However, since many people with depression also suffer from sleeping problems, these drugs work great to treat both problems at once (Suni, 2020c).

- **Anticonvulsants:** The next prescribed medication that you might encounter is an anticonvulsant. Anticonvulsants are drugs that are primarily used to treat seizures. However, off the label, it is often used to treat sleeping problems. Anticonvulsants contain anti-anxiety properties, which cause drowsiness in some people and can lead to better sleep. Research on using this type of drug to treat sleeping disorders is limited and, therefore, not the first course of action that doctors take unless you already suffer from seizures as well.

- **Antipsychotics:** The final prescribed medication that you need to be aware of is an antipsychotic drug. Antipsychotics are drugs that are used to treat patients with mental health disorders when the goal is to reduce their delusions and hallucinations. However, antipsychotics can be used to treat sleeping problems since they have a sedative effect due to the way that they can influence the chemical serotonin in the brain, which contributes to sleep quality. This also won't be most doctors' first approach to treating your sleeping disorder unless you show symptoms of hallucinations and feel delusional about certain aspects of your life (Suni, 2020c).

In general, prescribed medication works better over a long period of time. While over-the-counter medication might have immediate effects, prescribed medication is better for lifelong use, and it might take your body a couple of weeks to get used to the new medication and adjust accordingly. It's important not to mess with your prescribed medication since it can cause addiction. It can also be very dangerous when mixed with alcohol or taken carelessly. Just like over-the-counter medication, there are certain risks to prescription medication.

Risks

It's essential that your healthcare provider talk to you about the potential side effects of prescription medication before you start taking it. In some cases, certain side effects are infrequent, but it's not impossible, which is why you should be aware of the symptoms. Depending on the type of prescription medication, you might experience different side effects or run the possibility of different risks. However, there are a few common side effects and risks that you can expect from most prescription medications.

- dizziness and lightheadedness
- headaches and migraines
- drowsiness
- diarrhea
- nausea
- allergic reactions
- hallucinations
- cognitive changes, which can lead to bizarre behavior
- memory loss
- performance problems
- habit formation and addiction

In some cases, you might also experience tremors, a dry mouth, and an irregular heartbeat. It's important to talk to your doctor as soon as you experience any side effects to assess whether the medication is working effectively or not. Oftentimes, it takes a couple of trials and errors to determine which medication would work best for your body. Be sure to get an accurate medical evaluation before you start consuming prescription medication.

Precautions to Keep in Mind

Even though prescription medication can be dangerous, we don't have to avoid it or live in fear when we're using it since there are a couple of precautions that we can implement to keep us on the straight and narrow. There are ten precautions that you should implement when you're consuming prescription medication to ensure that you are not at risk of hurting yourself.

1. Before you start taking any medication, get approval from your doctor. Trust their professional judgment, and remember that they are the experts, not you.
2. Share which current medications you're taking with your doctor since different medications respond to each other differently.
3. Notify your doctor as soon as you experience any side effects, such as high blood pressure or an allergic reaction.
4. Read the package insert that comes with the medication to familiarize yourself with what are considered normal side effects and which ones are more serious. This will also help you understand what it is that you're taking.

5. Follow your prescription exactly as prescribed by the doctor. Don't increase or decrease your dosage on your own.

6. Avoid alcohol near the time when you are taking sleeping medication to avoid possible risks.

7. Only take a sleeping pill when you have a full night's rest ahead of you. Avoid drinking medication when you only have a couple of hours to sleep since the pill won't be "finished" working by the time you have to wake up, which can be dangerous.

8. Take the first dose on a night when you don't have to go anywhere the next morning so you can evaluate how you're feeling the next morning without the pressure of having to be somewhere.

9. Never drive anywhere after you've consumed a sleeping pill since that can be dangerous for you and the other cars on the road.

10. If you experience problems with taking the medication or are reluctant to take it, contact your doctor immediately and share your concerns with them.

Besides these ten rules, there is one more guideline that you should never forget, and that is that you should never hand out your prescription medication to others who you think might need it as well. Rather, encourage them to go to the doctor themselves and get their own prescription. If you haven't been struggling with your sleep for a long time and it's not necessarily as serious as the disorders we've discussed in this chapter, consider using an over-the-counter medication first. However, if your sleeping disorder is long-term and is affecting your life, it's essential that you seek medical attention right away. It's also important to know that medication isn't the only treatment for sleeping disorders, which is exactly what we'll be discussing in the next chapter.

The Best Gift You Can Share With Others is A Great Night's Sleep!

"Never waste any time you can spend sleeping."

— *FRANK H. KNIGHT*

If you have insomnia or a sleep disorder like sleep apnea, it can feel like you've landed on a strange planet where every waking hour is a struggle for survival. Your brain feels "fried," your skin looks tired, and you are worried about zoning out or falling asleep while driving, working, or spending time with loved ones.

Sleep deprivation goes way beyond daily professional and personal conundrums, of course. By this stage in your reading, you are well aware of the wide gamut of effects it has on so many bodily systems. Poor sleep is linked to stress, obesity, heart disease, and even Type 2 diabetes. Still, it is something that millions of people do not prioritize because other worries—their job and myriad of responsibilities—are always number one.

If you are reading this, then you have already taken the first, big step toward getting a restful night's sleep. We now have debunked myths like "Taking a nap stops you from sleeping at night." You have also discovered 5 easy yet powerful lifestyle changes that will very quickly make a big difference to the quantity and quality of your ZZZs.

If this book has enlightened you on the vital role your own choices play in achieving a restful sleep, I hope I can ask you to leave an honest opinion of the areas it has helped you most with.

Your review on Amazon will shed light for other readers who simply want nothing more than to sleep through the night and wake up feeling rested. Through your experience with the 10-tactic sleep program, you can show other readers that poor sleep is most definitely NOT "just another everyday problem."

You will let them know that the right quantity and quality of sleep will not only enhance their well-being but also add years to their life—and stave off chronic disease.

Your words will help them discover that they can, once more, know the bliss of sleeping like a baby. And they can start doing so in just a few days.

Scan this QR code to leave a review!

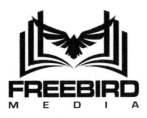

5

ALTERNATIVE TREATMENTS

D o you remember when I shared my story at the beginning of this book and how the sleep apnea mask literally saved my life and transformed my sleep? Well, others might experience the mask a little differently than I do. While for me, the mask signified freedom and good sleep, for others, it felt like a trap or a constriction. In fact, 40% of people diagnosed with obstructive sleep apnea find the mask treatment absolutely uncomfortable and unbearable (Cleveland Clinic, 2021). This is especially true for people who might suffer from claustrophobia. In some cases, the mask can lead to increased feelings of anxiety, which isn't something we want to experience when we're already struggling to fall asleep! Luckily, there are many other alternative treatments that we can use to treat sleeping disorders. What worked for me might not work for you at all, and that's totally okay! There isn't just one right answer; rather, you need to find the right answer for yourself, which might not be applicable to others.

In this chapter, we'll explore the different avenues of treatment for sleeping disorders. While some people don't mind being half-robot when they go to bed (like me and my Darth Vader helmet), others prefer a more natural approach. There are mainly five alternative treatment methods that we'll be discussing, as well as seven medical devices and therapies for people with sleep apnea specifically. We'll also look at the different benefits that the different treatments might have for you as well as the possible cons. Are you ready to learn all about alternative treatments other than medications? Then dive right in!

ALTERNATIVE TREATMENTS FOR SLEEP DISORDERS

If medication is not a route you want to explore, that's totally okay and understandable. There are many alternative treatments that can help with sleep disorders, and some basic life changes that you can implement to improve your sleep, as we discussed in Chapter 3. Even though there isn't a lot of scientific proof that other

SICK AND TIRED | 119

treatments can help, the proof is in the pudding, and I've met a lot of people who swear by these treatment plans. In this section, we'll specifically discuss five alternative treatments, which include

- acupuncture
- herbs
- CBD and cannabis
- sleep hypnosis
- light exposure

Acupuncture

Acupuncture is a traditional Chinese medicine that is used for the treatment of insomnia. Acupuncture consists of small needles that are inserted into the skin at specific points that influence the body (Begum, 2023). Acupuncture is a common treatment for insomnia but can also be used for other sleeping disorders. How and where the needles are inserted can influence how your body functions, and it can help you relax. Acupuncture helps you achieve better sleep quality since it increases pressure relief in your body. Acupuncture is often used alongside herbal treatments and electrical stimulation. The most obvious con of acupuncture is that it can be quite sore and uncomfortable to endure. It can also cause bruising, and in some cases, it can even cause bleeding. If you are on any medication that is considered a blood thinner, it's essential that you stay away from acupuncture since it can be very dangerous. When you use acupuncture, make sure that the practitioner is certified and that the needles are sterilized (Zwarensteyn, 2022).

Herbal Treatment

Herbs are the most natural and safest way to treat insomnia and other sleeping disorders. Herbs can either be taken as a tea or as a pill supplement. Even though herbs are safe, certain herbs might react strangely to medications you're already using, so it's best to run them past your healthcare provider to ensure the safety of the herbs and the other medications you're using. Ashwagandha is an herb that contains trimethylene glycol, which highly affects REM sleep. When you take about 300 milligrams of Ashwagandha a day, you will experience a higher quality of sleep. Chamomile is another herb that is quite well-known and loved. It can be used as a sleeping agent, and it can help you increase your sleep quality. However, it's essential to note that people with a ragweed allergy might also be allergic to chamomile. One of the biggest pros of using herbs to combat your sleep disorder is that they are easy to use. Most herbs can be found without a prescription and are sold at most health-related shops. There aren't any serious cons to herbal treatment, except if you're a child or pregnant. People with liver problems should also steer clear of herbal treatments.

CBD and Cannabis

Another alternative treatment method for sleep disorders is using CBD and Cannabis. CBD is short for cannabidiol, and it's a compound in cannabis without the psychoactive effects (the high). CBD and cannabis will help you fall asleep faster, but depending on where you live, it might be illegal to use them for sleep deprivation. As with other drugs, your brain will get used to CBD, and you will build a tolerance over time, meaning that you will have to increase your dosage if you want to see the same effects. That's why CBD is probably not an ideal solution for long-term use. There isn't enough research just yet about the effects of CBD usage on your sleep quality when used over a long period of time. CBD and cannabis are often viewed as unconventional treatments for insomnia and other sleeping disorders. However, many people claim that CBD helps them not only to fall asleep but also to stay asleep for the duration of the night (Zwarensteyn, 2022).

Sleep Hypnosis

Sleep hypnosis is a type of hypnotherapy that should be done only by a professional, which includes a psychologist, a doctor, or another healthcare provider who can guide you through it. Sleep Hypnosis makes use of a trance-like state of sleep where your licensed professional will work with you and suggest sleep-related changes as discussed with you while you are awake. The changes aim to address the underlying and subconscious sleep issues that you might have, such as anxiety (Zwarensteyn, 2022). There are a couple of common disadvantages to sleep hypnosis, which is why many people are hesitant to try this form of treatment. You might also experience a headache, dizziness, and false memories once the hypnosis is complete. Even though side effects fade quickly, it can still be a daunting process. However, there are no long-term side effects of sleep hypnosis, which makes it one of the safest alternative treatment solutions. It's essential that if you make use of this treatment style, you work with a licensed professional and not anyone else since hypnosis can be dangerous.

Light Exposure

The final alternative treatment method we should look at is light exposure therapy. This therapy is also known as phototherapy, which occurs when you are exposed to a light source that is brighter than the usual indoor light (Zwarensteyn, 2022). The light is ultimately brighter than direct sunlight, and it's easy to use. This method is prevalent among insomnia patients, and they use it every day at the same time for the same length of time to ensure the best results. Light exposure can also be used to treat depression, jet lag, and seasonal affective disorder. Since light affects your brain chemicals and is closely connected to your mood, your sleep will improve due to light exposure. However, light exposure can lead to an abnormal circadian rhythm, so you should consult your doctor before implementing any light exposure techniques into your life. If you have problems with your eyesight, they might be aggravated by light exposure, which can be pretty dangerous. Other illnesses, such as Lupus, can also worsen due to light exposure, and people with epilepsy should be careful when making use of this treatment (Zwarensteyn, 2022).

Even though these five alternative methods are commonly accepted in the US as treatment methods, it's essential that you speak to your doctor before starting them. It's also important that you keep track of the side effects and stop the treatment when you experience an increase in side effects such as vomiting, rapid heartbeat, anxiety, and skin rashes. When you use herbal treatments, be cautious of any product that mixes more than two herbs together, and be careful not to believe every commercial claim that they put on the box. Do some research first, and choose the brand carefully.

MEDICAL DEVICES FOR SLEEP APNEA

Besides the alternative treatments, there are a couple of medical devices that you can use when you specifically struggle with sleep apnea. A sleep apnea device won't cure your insomnia so be sure that you only make use of these devices once you are correctly diagnosed with sleep apnea. There are a couple of devices that you can use, and when choosing which one you want to invest in, it's essential that you know how each device works and what it is best used for. In this section, we'll look at seven different medical devices that can aid in your sleep apnea. Each device naturally comes with its own set of pros and cons, which we'll explore in closer detail. When choosing a medical device, it's crucial that you discuss the options with your healthcare provider and that you also take their advice into account (Ott, 2022).

CPAP Machine

CPAP stands for Continuous Positive Airway Pressure, which supplies and maintains the same pressure when you inhale and exhale. In other words, it holds your airway open when you're sleeping, which allows you to breathe properly (Ott, 2022). A CPAP machine is about the size of a small stereo and uses a tube that supplies air to the masks. Yes, I know it sounds like something out of a science fiction novel, and you're not far from wrong. Some of the latest CPAP machines have built-in humidifiers that ensure that the constant air isn't dry. CPAP machines have adjustable pressure features that allow you to breathe more naturally. Even though CPAP machines have many features to ensure comfort, some people find them very uncomfortable and not approachable at all. It might take some time to get used to the CPAP machine, but once you adjust to it, the benefits far outweigh the discomfort (Ott, 2022).

Pros of a CPAP machine include

- incredible in treating obstructive sleep apnea
- contains many comfort features to ensure that you are comfortable when you're sleeping
- you wake up feeling refreshed and alert
- it can pair with an app, which then tracks your sleep so you can see how much better the quality of sleep you're getting is
- it's available in various sizes, so you can travel with it

Cons of a CPAP machine include

- it can be pretty expensive
- it can be hard to adjust to the machine
- you might experience side effects like dry and itchy skin and mask soreness
- it can be uncomfortable to tolerate the pressure in the mask

As you read in my sleep story, a CPAP machine literally changed my life and helped me breathe normally and get a good quality of sleep. I would highly recommend this machine to anyone suffering from sleep apnea. There are also different types of CPAP machines that you can choose from:

- **Nasal Pillow:** This device creates a seal at the base of your nostrils. It's the least invasive mask, and it is recommended for men with facial hair. The nasal pillow doesn't provide a lot of pressure, so if your sleep apnea is severe, this might not be the best CPAP machine for you.
- **Face Mask:** The face mask seals around your nose and mouth. The mask is attached to four-point headgear that keeps the mask in place.

- **Face Mask with Chin Strap:** This mask is like a nasal pillow but with a chin strap to ensure that it's secure on your face.

APAP Machine

APAP machines are similar to CPAP machines. The most significant difference between the CPAP and the APAP machines is the pressure (Ott, 2022). While CPAP machines use constant pressure, the APAP machine provides just enough pressure to keep the airway open, making it more bearable. Some CPAP machines come with the ability to be APAP machines as well but at an additional cost. Other than that, an APAP, and a CPAP work virtually the same way. The APAP is beneficial since it adapts to your needs as your lifestyle changes. A CPAP requires recalibration when your prescription changes, while an APAP adjusts your needs automatically. The APAP is more personalized and can create a better course of treatment for you personally. The APAP machine is best for those who can't tolerate the CPAP machine but need it to open their airway and for people with a lot of allergies and flu-like symptoms (Ott, 2022).

The benefits of the APAP machine include

- it adjusts to your needs on a breath-by-breath basis
- equally as effective as the CPAP machine
- more comfortable than the CPAP machine
- available in travel-sized machines

Cons of the APA machine include

- even more expensive than the CPAP machine
- shares most of the cons of a CPAP machine

BiPAP Machine

A BiPAP is another machine that can be used to manage the pressure in your airway. A BiPAP is a two-way airway pressure machine that uses the same tubing as a CPAP or APAP machine. However, a BiPAP has two distinct pressure settings, one for inhaling and one for exhaling (Ott, 2022). This makes the BiPAP machine the perfect option for people with complicated breathing disorders that require a significant difference between inhaling and exhaling. In general, a BiPAP machine has the same minimum pressure setting as an APAP machine, but it can reach a much higher maximum than the APAP or CPAP machines. A BiPAP machine is perfect for those who have been diagnosed with a neurological condition that disrupts breathing and for people living with moderate to severe lung conditions. The BiPAP is also great for people who have been diagnosed with Obesity and hypoventilation syndrome (Ott, 2022).

Pros of the BiPAP machine include

- it uses the same hose and mask as APAP and CPAP
- it has a much higher pressure setting
- uses a distinct exhale and inhale pressure
- has the same comfort features as the APAP and CPAP models

Cons of the BiPAP machine include

- even more expensive than the APAP machine
- has the same drawbacks as the APAP and CPAP machines

Oral Appliances

Oral appliances are tools used to treat sleep apnea in an effective way that doesn't require you to tolerate air pressure. Oral appliances usually come in two types: The first is called a tongue-retaining device, which shields your tongue from creating a vacuum seal and keeps your tongue from falling back into the airway, blocking your airflow (Ott, 2022). The second is a mandibular advancement device (MAD), which treats sleep apnea by holding the jaw forward in an attempt to prevent the tongue from blocking your airway. A prescription is required for oral appliances, and they can't be bought over the counter. However, similar devices that are created to prevent snoring can be bought over the counter (Ott, 2022). Oral appliances are best for those with mild OSA and adults who have difficulty adapting to a CPAP machine. It is also good for children who struggle with obstructive sleep apnea:

Pros of oral appliances include

- it is effective in treating sleep apnea
- it is much more affordable
- it requires fewer lifestyle changes
- they can be readjusted as needed
- it doesn't require any electricity

Cons of oral appliances include

- it can worsen the symptoms of sleep apnea when not used properly
- it can be uncomfortable and might take some time to get used to
- may cause jaw stiffness

- it only lasts about 1 to 3 years before requiring a replacement

Hypoglossal Nerve Stimulation

A hypoglossal nerve stimulation device is a small device that is surgically implanted. It is implanted into your chest, and it aids in decreasing sleep apnea symptoms by electrically stimulating your hypoglossal nerve (Ott, 2022). Your hypoglossal nerve runs from your chest to your tongue, and it controls the muscles that move forward and backward in your tongue. The job of the nerve stimulator is to monitor your breathing, and when it detects an irregularity, it signals the nerve to control the chest and tongue muscles, helping you to keep your airway open in order to breathe. The hypoglossal nerve stimulator is perfect for people who have been diagnosed with moderate to severe OSA and those who have tried using a CPAP but didn't find it successful. It's also perfect for those who can't tolerate sleeping with a mask and those whose main issue is the obstruction of the tongue (Ott, 2022):

Pros of hypoglossal nerve stimulation include

- it can be turned on and off with a remote
- the device responds automatically, so you don't have to manage it

- it is safe and effective

Cons of the hypoglossal nerve stimulator include

- it requires a minimally invasive procedure
- it can be extremely expensive
- it only works if the obstruction is caused by the tongue
- it can become infected and require removal
- it's not recommended when you're pregnant or planning on becoming pregnant
- the battery will need replacement after 11 years

EPAP Valves

EPAP stands for Expiratory Positive Airway Pressure, which is a small device that gets inserted into your nostrils (Ott, 2022). The EPAP uses the pressure of your natural exhales to hold the airway open between breaths. The EPAP doesn't require a machine, and it doesn't supply pressure for you. It simply uses your natural breathing pressure to treat sleep apnea. The EPAP is less likely to make a patient feel claustrophobic, and it's super easy to stick with it long-term. The EPAP is highly recommended to anyone who struggles to adjust to the CPAP and if you're a frequent traveler since it transports much easier than other machines. It's also a perfect solution for anyone who has limited access to electricity since it doesn't require a motor or battery (Ott, 2022):

Pros of the EPAP Valve include

- it's more affordable than other devices
- it doesn't require any electricity to work
- portable
- better compliance than the CPAP machine

Some of the cons of the EPAP valve include

- it doesn't work for everybody
- not ideal to treat severe sleep apnea
- not quite as effective as the CPAP

Position Pillows

A positioning pillow is a device that keeps you from turning onto your back when you're sleeping. Moderate sleep apnea can be effectively treated by addressing the sleeping position and preventing sleeping on the back. However, position therapy isn't quite as effective as the CPAP machine, and since it only treats moderate sleep apnea, it's not suited for everyone. There is a wide range of position pillows that people can try out to see if they relieve their sleep apnea symptoms (Ott, 2022).

- CPAP pillow, which is designed for those already using a CPAP mask. The pillow supports different sleeping positions by using divots and cutouts to naturally accommodate the equipment of the CPAP.
- Wedge pillows elevate your lower body from the waist up, which helps relieve the gravitational pressure. These pillows are very helpful with acid reflux and GERD symptoms.
- Side sleeping pillows are full-body pillows that help position your body in such a way that your tongue can't collapse into your airway.

Position therapy is best used for those who only experience mild sleep apnea symptoms or those who already use other devices. If you're on a budget, position pillows are the most cost-effective route to take. Position pillows are also great for people who are unable to undergo invasive therapies like hypoglossal nerve stimulation. The pros of the position pillows include

- it is customizable, and there are different options to choose from
- it's inexpensive
- can ease other symptoms like GERD and acid reflux
- it's a non-committal treatment option

- it can be combined with other treatments

The cons of position pillows include

- it's not as effective as the CPAP machine
- it's not guaranteed to bring relief
- it doesn't help those whose airways are blocked by excessive tissue

Now that you have a better idea of the alternative treatments available for you and a clear picture of the different medical devices that can be used to treat sleep apnea, it's important to talk to your doctor before making any decisions. In some cases, sleeping disorders resolve fairly quickly after a couple of weeks, but in other cases, people might not be as lucky and struggle for years. In the next chapter, we'll look at how to manage sleep disorders that last longer than just a couple of weeks and how to prepare yourself for long-term sleep disorders.

6

MANAGING SLEEP DISORDERS
LONG TERM

When I'm worried and I can't sleep, I count my blessings instead of sheep.

— IRVING BERLIN

There is a secret weapon for managing sleep disorders that not many people talk about. In fact, it's one of those secret weapons that are often overlooked when you have access to them, but as soon as they're removed, you feel the consequences heavily. The secret weapon I'm referring to is the power of a support system. Managing a sleep disorder over the long-term can be incredibly taxing on your system and managing it all on your own is even worse. It can make you feel isolated, lonely, and like an onlooker in your own life. However, with a support system, everything is a little bit easier.

When I was first diagnosed with sleep apnea, I was a little embarrassed. I didn't want to tell people about it, and I was so self-conscious that I didn't want to sleep next to my wife. For a couple of months, I hid it pretty well, but then we got invited to go away for a weekend with a group of friends. This trip was an annual thing, so I agreed to join our friends before really thinking about what that would mean. When the time came to start packing, I tried my best to hide my mask and machine, but no matter how I tried, I couldn't get them to fit into my suitcase. Eventually, I gave up and just hid it under my jacket. Of course, the jacket fell off right as we arrived and revealed my big, dark secret to everyone.

At first, I pretended like nothing happened, but then my friends started asking questions. Even though I was embarrassed, we shared our journey with them and explained the severity of the situation. While I was scared it would alienate me; my friends were extremely supportive. They asked how they could help, and they offered up their time and energy to support me and my family. What I thought would be embarrassing turned out to be a big blessing! It felt like a weight had been lifted off my shoulders! That's the beauty of a support system.

I know you might be tempted to go on this journey alone and figure things out for yourself, but I really want to encourage you to find yourself a support system and allow others to be there for you. In this chapter, we'll discuss the power of a support system as well as how you can support those around you. We'll also look at ways that you can manage your sleep disorder at work and how to deal with long-distance traveling while suffering from a sleep disorder. All of this will help you manage long-term sleeping disorders.

HOW TO SUPPORT OTHERS

Perhaps you're not the only one with a sleeping disorder in your inner circle. Maybe one of your friends or a family member also suffers from a sleeping disorder, and you're not sure how to support them. Or maybe you want support from your family and friends, but you're not sure how they can help. In this section, we'll look at ways to support others who are suffering from a sleeping disorder. You can also use these tips to ask for similar support. You can ask others to support you in this way while also learning how to support others. It's incredibly hard to go about your day when you are entirely sleep-deprived, which is why having support is so vital. Let's have a look at seven ways that you can support others with sleep disorders or how your support system can help you (The Recovery Village, 2022).

Encouragement to Journal

The first way that you can help others, or how others can help you, is by encouraging the person with the sleeping disorder to start a sleeping journal. The goal of a sleeping journal is to provide yourself with data to analyze. Since it might be necessary to go to a health-care provider, having data that shows your sleeping patterns will significantly speed up the process and help you find a healthy solution for your sleeping disorder. Starting a sleeping journal is a great way of getting to the root of the issue, and it can include all sorts of sleep-related journal entries. For example, you can write down what you ate for dinner and at what time. You can note when you went to bed and what bedtime routine you followed. You can also write down how you felt in the morning, whether you had intense dreams, and whether you woke up a lot during the night. The more detail you provide, the better you'll be able to start noticing patterns of what might work and what might not (The Recovery Village, 2022).

Other things that you can include in the journal are

- what time you woke up
- the quality of the sleep you had
- how much time you spent awake
- how long it took you to fall asleep
- your daily physical activity
- your thoughts and feelings
- your mood throughout the day

Check-in on Their Sleep

Another way that you can support others or ask to be supported is by checking in on your partner's sleep. Since some people struggle with sleep apnea, they might stop breathing at night and not be aware of it. Just like how I was completely oblivious to the fact that I stopped breathing frequently, your loved one might also be unaware of the severity of the situation. Checking in on their sleep doesn't mean that you have to watch them sleep every minute. Rather, when you wake up to go to the bathroom or for other reasons, check in on them and watch to see if you notice anything out of the ordinary. You can also ask a loved one to specifically wake up one night to watch you sleep and check for any abnormalities (The Recovery Village, 2022). This will give you a clear picture of whether you're suffering from sleep apnea or something else.

Listen

The biggest benefit of having a support system is having someone who listens to you. As human beings, we don't always want advice! I remember sharing my frustration with a friend once about how tired I felt, and suddenly, I got bombarded with a list of things that I should do to improve my sleep, followed by their testimony of how incredibly rested they were. I was so annoyed that I just got up and walked away. Later that day, I met up with another friend. At first, I was hesitant to share, but after they specifically asked about my sleep disorder, I frustratingly shared how tired I felt. Instead of giving solutions to the problem, they just listened to me vent. Eventually, they said, "That sucks. I'm so sorry!" That made me feel better. Knowing that others understood that it wasn't easy and that it really sucked sometimes was all I really wanted that day. I just wanted someone to listen to me, and I'm so thankful for that listening friend. Be sure to listen to your loved ones when they share their frustrations with you. Don't always jump to a solution; first, just listen and offer support in that way.

Establish a Routine

Having a bedtime routine is essential when treating sleeping disorders, but it can be quite hard to establish and maintain a bedtime routine on your own. If you live with a loved one who's experiencing a sleep disorder, one of the best ways that you can support them is by creating a bedtime routine together. Establishing a routine together will improve relaxation and promote healthy sleeping habits. So, what can your bedtime routine include? You can start by enjoying a cup of herbal tea after you both have showered and put away all your devices. Once your tea is finished, you can practice a breathing exercise together or meditate for a couple of minutes. You can then end the day by journaling together about your current state of mind. When you establish a routine together, the person struggling with the sleeping disorder will feel supported and encouraged to maintain the new routine, and it can also bring you and your loved one closer together. If you're the one struggling with a sleeping disorder, you can invite a loved one to join you in your bedtime routine and create one together. You don't have to wait for someone else to create the bedtime routine for you (The Recovery Village, 2022).

Create a Comfortable Environment

Your sleep environment contributes significantly to the quality of your sleep. One way that you can support a loved one with a sleeping disorder is by helping them create a comfortable sleeping environment. Whether that means investing in black-out curtains or perhaps helping them to declutter their bedroom, every little thing contributes to the overall success. You can also suggest that they experiment with white noise or perhaps even with room temperature. If it's your partner that's struggling with sleep, be supportive in trying out new possible fixes without complaining about it keeping you awake. Instead, work together to find something that would work for both of you. If you're the one with sleeping problems, you can ask for your partner's support by brainstorming ideas to elevate the comfort of your bedroom together (The Recovery Village, 2022).

Reduce Their Stress

Stress contributes to all sleep disorders, so it's incredibly helpful when you find a way to reduce stress in your loved one's life. Whether that's by taking over some of their responsibilities or by encouraging them to destress daily, you can help them reduce their stress levels. You can start by making sure that your home is a stress-free zone. Make sure that your environment is relaxing and comfortable. You can help your loved ones get rid of stress, not only before bed but during the day. Activities such as yoga and meditation are great ways to release some stress. You can also encourage your loved one to take a couple of days off from work or to help them create healthy boundaries at work to reduce stress. By helping your loved one reduce stress, you will also be reducing your own stress levels. If you're the one struggling with sleeping disorders, you can ask your loved ones for support by asking them to remove some of the stressors from your life. You can start by asking a loved one to take care of dinner instead of having to worry about it. Reducing stress isn't difficult, but it needs to be intentional if you want it to be effective.

Encourage Them to Seek Treatment

The final way that you can support a loved one who is struggling with a sleeping disorder is by encouraging them to seek treatment. Often, we are reluctant to seek treatment because we're unsure what to expect. We're scared of the outcome and worried about how it might influence the rest of our lives. It's essential that you support your loved one by explaining to them that seeking treatment is a good idea and that it doesn't make you "weird." In fact, when you seek treatment, it shows a great deal of courage. Since many sleep disorders can lead to mental issues, it's good to seek treatment both physically and mentally. If you're the one struggling with sleeping problems, talk to a loved one and ask their advice on treatment. Explain your thinking process and ask them to support you in finding the correct type of treatment for your sleeping disorder (The Recovery Village, 2022). When you start treatment, you will need a support system to help you adjust to the new changes in your life.

Supporting a friend or a family member can feel awkward at first, and you might be scared of not knowing what to do or say, but it's important that you show others that you are there for them and that you want to help in any way that you can. In the next section, we'll look at how we can find help from others and which specialists to contact for different needs.

FINDING HELP IN OTHERS

Despite getting all the love and support from friends and family, sometimes we need external help to manage our sleeping disorder, especially when it lasts for a long time. Different specialists can help us with different sleeping disorders, and it's important to know who to seek help from and when. In this section, we'll look at the different medical specialists that can help with sleeping disorders and who to seek out first. One of the easiest ways to find help from a specialist is by speaking to your healthcare provider and asking for a referral. You can also ask friends and family if they know anyone that they would recommend.

The different areas of expertise include the following (Watson, 2020a):

- **Psychiatrists:** Since many sleep disorders are rooted in fear and anxiety, speaking to a psychiatrist will help you to clear out your head and let go of the thoughts and behaviors that are causing the sleep problems. When your sleep disorder is rooted in trauma or being burned out, seeking help from a psychiatrist is the best course of action since it won't just treat the symptoms but get to the root of the problem.
- **Neurologists:** A neurologist treats the nervous system, which is why they are very helpful when you're suffering from central sleep apnea. With sleep apnea, your brain fails to send the correct signals to the rest of your body to control your breathing. So, a neurologist can help you pinpoint the issue and work with you to find the proper treatment to correct the brain's signals.

- **Pediatricians:** Pediatricians work closely with children, so if you have a child that needs help with sleeping disorders, a pediatrician is the best course of action (Watson, 2020a).
- **Otorhinolaryngologists:** When you are suffering from obstructive sleep apnea, an otorhinolaryngologist will help you find the right treatment. An otorhinolaryngologist specializes in ear, nose, and throat issues and is often revered as an ear, nose, and throat specialist. The specialists will be able to check to see if you have any blockages in your nose and throat, and they'll be able to prescribe the best course of action for you personally.
- **Dentists:** In some cases, you might need an oral appliance to correct the problem in your mouth that is causing your sleeping disorder. That's where dentists come in. The dentist will be able to fit you with an oral appliance that will work best for you and correct the problem in your mouth and jaw.
- **Pulmonologists:** A pulmonologist specializes in the lungs and can prescribe medical devices that will help you breathe at night, like a CPAP machine. A pulmonologist can also diagnose you with other sleep conditions that could be affecting your sleep, such as chronic obstructive

pulmonary disease. A pulmonologist can help you find the solution to your sleeping disorder when the problem is caused by the lungs.

- **Cardiologists:** Many sleeping disorders are linked to high blood pressure, irregular heartbeats, heart failure, and stroke. A cardiologist can diagnose and treat all of these heart-related issues as part of your sleep apnea care. A cardiologist will also be able to help you find the best course of action to take special care of your heart health, which contributes to longevity.

WHEN TO SEE A SPECIALIST

Knowing who to see is only one piece of the puzzle. I've found that people struggle more often with *when* to seek help from a specialist than with *who* to seek help from. I would suggest seeking help from a specialist as soon as you think you might have a sleeping disorder. If you often wake up gasping for air or if you snore a lot, take these as signs that you might need some sleeping help. You can also seek help from a specialist if you struggle to fall or stay asleep at night. If this only happens once in a while, it's worth looking at your habits first, but if it's a common occurrence, take it as a sign to seek help from a specialist. Another sign that it might be time to see a specialist is if you are increasingly tired during the day, even if you slept the night before. This can be due to many reasons, but it's best to have it checked out by those who are trained to do so. Finally, whenever you are so tired that you can't even do your daily tasks or participate in daily activities, it's time to seek external help from a specialist. If you're not sure whether it's serious enough to seek the help of a sleep specialist, visit your primary care doctor first and hear their opinion on the matter. Struggles with sleep can influence not only your personal life but also your work life, which is why it's essential to manage it effectively when you can. Let's take a look at how we can cope with a sleeping disorder at work.

COPING WITH A SLEEP DISORDER AT WORK

Did you know that about 20% of working adults work irregular shifts at work? That means that they work outside of the typical nine-to-five workday. Nontraditional work hours can be a big plus for some people, but in many cases, they can lead to a circadian rhythm sleep disorder known as Shift Work Sleep Disorder (Gupta, 2023). Working in shifts might be due to working in the public health and safety domain, which requires 24-hour operations. But why does working in shifts influence us so much if we still get 8 hours of sleep, just not during the night? Well, that's because our bodies have a 24-hour cycle that is attuned to the sun. When the sun goes down, our circadian rhythm is triggered, which governs our sleep, digestion, blood pressure, heart rate, and hormone production. In other words, we are programmed to sleep when it's dark and wake up when it's light. When you work night shifts, you mess with your rhythm and interfere with how your body usually works.

There are many symptoms of shift work sleep disorder, and many of these might even correspond with other sleeping disorder symptoms. These symptoms include (Gupta, 2023):

- feeling chronically fatigued
- constantly feeling irritated
- decreased alertness
- having trouble concentrating
- struggling to function in daily tasks
- impaired memory
- excessive daytime sleepiness
- experiencing nightmares
- struggling to fall and stay asleep

When you struggle with shift work sleep disorder, you also open yourself up to many serious mental and physical health issues. When you work irregular hours, you raise your risk of cancer, stroke, heart disease, infertility, diabetes, hormonal imbalance, digestive issues, and obesity (Gupta, 2023). It can also lead to depression and anxiety, which in turn worsen the other symptoms. So, what can we do about it? It's not like we should suddenly close hospitals at night or tell firefighters that they're not allowed to do their job when it's still dark! That would create even more madness. However, there are a couple of things that we can do to cope with shift work disorder appropriately without letting anyone down or totally destroying our health and careers.

Let's have a look at a couple of ways that we can cope with shift work sleep disorder (Gupta, 2023):

- **Regulate Light Exposure:** You can regulate light exposure by keeping bright lights on while you're on your night shift. This can help you stay awake since it resembles sunlight. When you get home, make sure to close all the curtains and switch off all the lights to make it as dark as possible while sleeping. You can also invest in black-out curtains to ensure that your room is as dark as possible when it's time for bed.
- **Prioritize Sleep:** When you're not on duty, make sure that you prioritize sleep and get enough rest. You can also make sure to stick to

sleeping at night, where possible, on your off days or when you're on vacation.

- **Solicit Family Members' Cooperation:** Make sure to keep your family and friends up to date with your schedule and ask them not to disturb you when you're sleeping. You can request that they use headphones or be quiet when you're sleeping after a night shift. You can also make sure that they know when you're sleeping so that they don't call you or show up at your house.

- **Don't Drive Tired:** Instead of driving when you're tired, make alternative arrangements. You can either call a cab, take public transportation, or ask a loved one to pick you up. When you drive when you're tired, you might force yourself awake, which will make it hard to fall asleep once you get home. Worst-case scenario; you are so tired that you fall asleep while driving, causing an accident and being a danger to yourself and those around you.

- **Plan Naps:** Most places where you work the night shift have sleeping spaces where you can take a nap. Be sure to plan your naps, if you can, while working night shifts and on a break. Try to rotate nap breaks with your coworkers over the course of the night shift to ensure that you get enough rest.

- **Avoid Rotating Shifts:** Where possible, avoid rotating shifts. Rather, work either during the day or during the night and try not to rotate between the two. When you rotate, you confuse your body even more, while when you don't rotate, you give your body time to settle into the new rhythm.

- **Use a Sleeping Aid:** If you struggle to fall asleep after a night shift, check in with your healthcare provider and ask for a sleeping aid such as melatonin. Work with a specialist if necessary to get you the right aid to ensure at least 8 hours of sleep.

- **Maintain a Healthy Routine:** Even if your days and nights are switched, it's essential that you maintain a healthy routine. Working shifts might make it hard to go to the gym or eat healthy meals, but it's important to follow a healthy routine and diet if you want to improve your immunity. So, prioritize sticking to a routine, even when it looks different than everyone else's.

Working in shifts can be incredibly hard, but it doesn't have to be dangerous to your health. By implementing these simple tips, you can prevent shift work sleep disorders and ensure that your sleep hygiene remains healthy and clean. Besides working in shifts, when you have to travel often, it can also highly influence your sleep hygiene. In the next section, we'll look at how traveling affects your sleep and how we can recover after traveling abroad and crossing time zones.

TRAVELING AND SLEEP

Before we jump right into the good stuff, we first need to address the elephant in the room. It's essential that you understand that there's a big difference between travel fatigue and being jet-lagged. Yes, I know, they sound the same, and in your mind, they might have merged into one idea, but it's actually not the same concept at all. Travel fatigue is when you feel temporarily exhausted when you're traveling. It can also include a headache and feeling slightly confused. Travel fatigue doesn't require crossing time zones, which is why it's different from jet lag. Jet lag is a temporary sleep problem that happens when you cross two or more time zones. Jet lag confuses your internal clock, and it affects your sleep since your body is still synced to the original time zone and not the time zone of your new location (American Thoracic Society, 2021). Jet lag can be pretty hard to cope with, but luckily there are some things that we can do to ease the side effects and prepare our bodies to adapt to the new time zone:

- **Adapt as quickly as possible:** As soon as you arrive in the new time zone, change your watch and other devices to accurately represent the time zone that you're in. Try your best to forget your old time zone, and don't compare the hours since that will only make you feel more tired. Try your best to sleep only once it's night in your new time zone, so eat meals and go to bed according to your new time zone and not the one you came from.

- **Manage your sleep:** Prioritize your new sleep schedule even when you're on the plane. If you know that it will be the night when you arrive, avoid sleeping while you're traveling and only sleep once you get there. If it's going to be morning when you arrive, try to sleep on the plane to ensure that you have enough energy to manage an entire day before sleeping. Earplugs and a comfortable pillow might just be what you need when you're sleeping on the plane, so make sure that you're comfortable and prepared to either sleep or stay awake intentionally.

- **Stay hydrated:** Long-distance traveling can cause dehydration, so make sure that you consume enough water while traveling. Proper hydration will also help manage the jet lag symptoms.
- **Light Exposure:** Since jet lag interrupts your internal clock, try light exposure once you've reached your new destination. If it's daytime, spend some time in the sun, and if it's nighttime, make sure you turn off all bright lights and devices.
- **Drink some caffeine:** Drinking coffee or other caffeinated beverages won't cure your jet lag, but it can help you stay awake and focused enough to adapt to the new time zone. If you know that you're losing time when flying and entering a new destination when it's nighttime, avoid drinking caffeinated beverages a couple of hours prior and steer clear of sugary foods.

One of these tips alone won't completely cure jet lag, but together they can ease the symptoms tremendously. After you've traveled and are back home, there are other tips and tricks that you can implement to reduce travel fatigue and jet lag. Let's have a look at how we can recover quickly and ensure good sleep hygiene once we're finished traveling.

HOW TO RECOVER AFTER TRAVELING

Have you ever traveled and gotten home more tired than you were when you left? Instead of feeling calm, rested, and refreshed, you feel grumpy, exhausted, and anything but ready for real life to return. Well, that's thanks to travel fatigue! Luckily, we have access to great resources and research that has found ways through which we can battle our travel fatigue. These things might seem silly and insignificant, but when done properly and together, they can quite literally transform you from feeling like the most tired person on earth to a refreshed person ready to take on the world! I encourage you to take notes as you're going through this section to ensure that you really grasp its importance:

- **Stay in one place:** When you're traveling long-term, you can prevent exhaustion by traveling slowly. Instead of rushing from one destination to the next, take your time and live like a local.
- **Take a nap:** Once you return home from traveling and it's still a while before sleeping again, take a short nap to get you through the night. However, make sure that you still get a proper night's sleep.

- **Eat fruits and veggies:** When you're traveling, you might be tempted to eat loads of fried food and treats. However, when you're traveling, it's essential that you still eat enough fruits and vegetables to ensure sound sleep and a healthy mind and body.
- **Unplug and meditate:** When you're able to recenter yourself and connect with your body, you will adapt to the change in routine and environment more easily. Make sure to recover from traveling by being present, unplugging from all distractions, and meditating on where you are and what you're feeling.
- **Exercise:** I know this might sound counterintuitive, but one of the best ways to recover after traveling is by exercising and moving. When you move your body, you increase your heart rate, which improves your sleeping habits.
- **Schedule time for recovery:** Once you get home, make sure you have a day or two to recover and adjust after the travels before having to go back to work. When you're traveling long distances, make sure that you also schedule recovery time once you arrive at the new destination.

Managing sleeping disorders long-term isn't impossible, but it will require you to be patient with yourself and to be intentional about prioritizing rest where possible. However, it's good news to know that it's not unmanageable. You can still do and experience everything that you want to, even while still struggling with your sleeping habits. Since a lot of sleeping disorders are connected to stress, you might even find that when you travel, you experience a decrease in your sleeping disorder symptoms. So, why not book a trip and start prioritizing your rest right away? There are also other advanced strategies that can help you manage your sleeping disorder long-term, which is exactly what we'll look at in the next chapter.

7

ADVANCED STRATEGIES

Have you ever had a nightmare where robots take over the world and destroy all human beings, or is that just me? Well, regardless of your answer, technology can be a great help to those of us struggling with sleep disorders. Even though, as a little boy, I feared having a robot who would take over the world; I am now so grateful that technology has evolved enough to address certain sleeping disorder issues. In this chapter, we'll explore the role of technology when it comes to sleep as well as specific devices that can improve overall sleep quality. We'll also discover other strategies, such as light therapy and cognitive behavioral therapy, and how they can contribute to our sleep health.

As they say, necessity is the mother of invention, and these advanced strategies surely prove how much society longs for good quality sleep and rest. Technology is molding our society, and thankfully, it's also improving our daily lives. Whether it's improving it by presenting a new business idea or by allowing us to have an advanced lifestyle, it's playing a role in our day-to-day activities. Technology is also improving our quality of life. In all honesty, who knows where I'd be today without my CPAP machine? I might have ended up dying in my sleep or still struggling to make it through the day with my eyes open. Technology has seeped into every area of our lives, and it's not all doom and gloom, as some people might think. Technology is also saving lives, literally, and it can also help you sleep better.

THE ROLE OF TECHNOLOGY

Since sleep plays such a big role in our lives, it is inevitable that technology will also find a way to improve it. One of the biggest ways that technology influences our sleep is through the use of apps. Sleep-tracking applications on your smartphone can help you keep track of your sleeping cycles and patterns. When you understand your sleeping cycles and patterns, you will have the knowledge to do something about them. You start to see where you need improvement and how you can achieve better-sleeping quality. There are hundreds of sleeping apps out there, but here are a few that I highly recommend:

- **Sleep as an Android:** If you're an Android user, this app is perfect for you. Sleep on Android is an alarm clock as well as a cycle tracker. What makes Sleep As Android so unique is the fact that it wakes you up when you're in the best cycle to be woken up. It doesn't wake you up while you're in a deep sleep like other alarm clocks. The app also includes other unique features that can help you elevate your sleep quality.
- **Jawbone Up:** The Jawbone Up fitness tracker comes paired with an app that also keeps track of your sleep, activities, and food. It also tracks your steps and measures the quality of your sleep. It even shows you how many times a day you fall asleep or how long you stay in bed before waking up. It's the perfect all-around tracker for both Android and iOS users.
- **Sleep Cycle:** Sleep Cycles track your sleep and the different cycles of sleep that you go

through. It also keeps track of the time that you spend awake, and you'll be able to see exactly how much deep sleep you get in a day. However, if you want this app to be accurate, you need to position your phone next to your head on your nightstand and not under a pillow. Sleep Cycle also records any sounds or movements that you make during the night.

- **MotionX-24/7:** This app is only available on iOS, and it correlates your heart rate to your sleep quality. This app uses your phone's camera to track your pulse from your fingertip. It monitors your sleep cycle, and it even provides you with features to help you fall asleep on nights when you're struggling.
- **Withings Health Mate:** This is another iOS-only app that works with an armband. It tracks your breathing and offers you personalized feedback.
- **Sleepbot:** The last app that I recommend is Sleepbot. The Sleepbot is a three-in-one app. It works as a smart alarm, a motion tracker, and a sound recorder. When you're about to go to bed, the app plays soothing music, which automatically stops once you're asleep.

Now, I know I mentioned earlier that you should try not to be on your phone at least an hour before bed, and that's still true. Even when you use a smart app to help you fall asleep, you don't have to be on your phone for the app to start working. You can set an automatic timer on your app. I suggest placing your phone face down so that no notification lights bother you when you're sleeping. Above all, remember that using an app to aid in your sleep is very different from scrolling on your phone on social media for hours before you go to sleep. So, be sure to use technology to your advantage and not your disadvantage.

TECHNOLOGICAL DEVICES THAT IMPROVE SLEEP

Besides apps, there are also other technological devices that contribute to better sleep quality. I know that having your smartphone track your sleep isn't for everyone, and that's perfectly okay. If you have no desire to track your sleep, then you don't have to. There are other ways to improve your sleep without the need for any apps. However, the combination of apps and these technological devices that we'll speak about now together form a powerful team to improve sleep quality. Let's take a look at six other devices that will most certainly improve your sleep in no time.

Smart Clocks

Smart clocks help you schedule enough hours of sleep per night. It will automatically limit your screen time on your phone when it's time to head to bed, and it will also send you reminders when it's time to turn off other distractions. Smart clocks can also play music to help you unwind at night and automatically stop the music after a couple of hours. Overall, smart clocks can help you manage your schedule better and improve the overall quality of your sleep (Alaska Sleep, 2022). Some smart clocks also prevent you from snoozing in the morning by prompting you with an activity you need to complete before turning off the alarm.

Temperature Control

A smart temperature control device, such as an automatic thermostat, controls the temperature in your room. Ultimately, it prevents your room from getting either too cold or too hot, which can both influence the quality of your sleep. In many cases, we might turn up the heat when we get into bed in order to fight the cold sheets, but as soon as we fall asleep, we'll feel too hot, and our sleep gets disturbed. A smart thermostat prevents this from happening by monitoring the temperature in your room and turning it on and off automatically to maintain that specific temperature.

This ensures high-quality sleep without having to get up in the middle of the night to adjust the temperature.

Interior Light Control

Since we already understand the importance of light on our circadian rhythm, it's no surprise to know that there are devices that can help control this. Automatic light bulbs will dim and emit less brightness as the day goes by. By evening, your lights won't be extremely bright but rather start to dim out slightly. It will adjust with the background to make sure that the house is still lit enough for you to see but not so light that it influences your circadian rhythm (Alaska Sleep, 2022). Lights that are adjustable are perfect for this since you can dim the lights in each room, you're in while someone in another room might still want brightness.

Blue Light Blockers

When you're exposed to blue light, it highly affects your circadian rhythm since it mimics the blue light of nature, signaling your brain and body to be awake and alert. Blue has the highest concentration of light and is therefore known as the color that keeps you awake. Exposure to blue light right before bed can disrupt your sleep cycle quite significantly. That's why blue-light blockers are such an incredible invention. Blue light blockers are built into most smart devices to ensure that your device dims as the night draws near. It will give your body time to adjust to nighttime and prepare for bed. You can also purchase blue light-blocking glasses, which reduce the intensity of all blue light and induce sleepiness (Alaska Sleep, 2022).

Relaxing Sounds and White Noise

Another great invention that can aid in the quality of your sleep is using devices that play relaxing sounds or white noise. Smart devices can play music and sounds that help your brain relax and eventually cause you to fall asleep. For some people, listening to the rain or a train running on a track is a sure ticket to good sleep, while other people enjoy soft nature music and birds. Sleep-time ambient music can prevent you from struggling to fall asleep by playing gentle music (Alaska Sleep, 2022). The repetition of gentle sounds causes your brainwaves to lower and your body to relax accordingly, resulting in great-quality sleep. If you haven't tried using a white noise machine, I highly recommend trying it for a night or two.

Smart Beds

The final smart device I want to talk about is a smart bed. Smart beds automatically adjust to provide comfort when you're sleeping. Smart beds have sensors that monitor your sleep and detect your temperature. It adjusts accordingly to provide you with an optimal environment that promotes quality sleep. The smart bed doesn't only focus on the temperature in the room; it also detects your temperature, ensuring even better temperature regulation than other thermostats (Alaska Sleep, 2022). The smart bed also gathers data regarding your breathing, heart rate, and the length of time that you spend in bed and actually sleeping. Of course, this device is naturally more expensive than the other devices, but it sure is an investment worth making.

These technological devices can contribute to the overall quality of your sleep tremendously. However, if you don't have the finances to invest in these technological devices or prefer other methods of treatment, there are other options as well. Advanced strategies aren't all about technology and sleep-inducing robots. In fact, some advanced strategies are quite ancient but still very relevant to our modern-day sleeping disorders. Two of the most common advanced therapies are light therapy and cognitive behavioral therapy.

LIGHT THERAPY

As we already know, there is a strong connection between sleep and light. Over the course of this book, we spoke about blocking out light quite a few times in order to ensure quality sleep. But did you know that light, at the right time, can also help you sleep better? Light therapy is designed to treat sleep conditions through exposure to artificial light (Pacheco, 2020). During a light therapy session, the patient will be positioned in front of a specialized device known as the light therapy box. The therapy box emits a bright light that is similar to natural sunlight. Light therapy is often used to treat patients with insomnia and other circadian rhythm sleep disorders. Light therapy can also be used for

- seasonal affective disorder
- depression
- jet lag
- working a night shift schedule
- Alzheimer's disease
- dementia

The science behind this therapy is quite straightforward. Being exposed to artificial light for a certain amount of time each day will bring your circadian rhythm back into the correct cycle. Depending on the severity of your disorder, the amount of light emitted will differ. The light triggers the production of melatonin and serotonin, which provide your body with a better sleep-wake cycle (Pacheco, 2020). Light has been found to be one of the most powerful tools for influencing your circadian rhythm. The best thing about light therapy is that you can also do it at home. There are many light therapy products that you can buy to aid in your sleeping disorder. Some of these products include

- table lamp
- floor lamp
- alarm clock
- wearable visor
- tablet-like device

These products are all relatively inexpensive and easily accessible. Not to mention that this type of therapy is also considered one of the safest types of therapy. However, like with most treatments, there are some possible side effects. If you have a skin or eye condition, this might not be the best course of action for you since the light might be too harsh on your body. Other people who are more likely to experience serious side effects are those who suffer from bipolar disorder. Even though this therapy can help lighten the effects of your sleeping disorder, it is not considered a cure (Pacheco, 2020).

COGNITIVE BEHAVIORAL THERAPY FOR INSOMNIA

Other than light therapy, another popular treatment can be found in Cognitive Behavioral Therapy for Insomnia (CBT-I). In short, this therapy is an evidence-based psychotherapy that is designed specifically to treat insomnia (St. Luke's Clinic, 2023). Instead of focusing on the side effects of insomnia, CBT-I focuses on treating the source of the insomnia. It specifically focuses on the feelings and beliefs that you might have about sleep and how they can negatively influence the quality of your sleep. Through this type of therapy, you have the opportunity to address your sleep patterns and retrain your mind to sleep when and where you need to. Usually, a CBT-I treatment consists of therapy sessions that last about 45 minutes. Most patients respond to CBT-I therapy relatively quickly and see results within a couple of sessions. CBT-I uses different kinds of instructions and procedures depending on each patient's specific needs. Let's have a closer look at a couple of these types of treatment in order to gain a better understanding of what CBT-I addresses.

Stimulus Control

The goal of stimulus control is to strengthen the cues for sleep and weaken the cues for wakefulness. It makes use of a set of instructions that address conditioned wakefulness. These instructions start by establishing a regular morning rise time in order to strengthen your circadian clock (Stanford Medicine, 2023). Within the instructions, you are also tasked with sticking to a regular bedtime in order to submit to your circadian rhythm. However, another instruction, especially for those struggling with insomnia, is to only go to bed once you are sleepy. Since the probability of falling asleep is much higher when you are already feeling sleepy, the goal is to make use of sleepiness (Stanford Medicine, 2023). If you are unable to fall asleep, stimulus control advises you to get up from bed and do something else until you feel sleepy again. Once you feel ready to sleep, you can return to bed once more. Stimulus control also advises against taking naps during the day and avoiding nocturnal sleep.

Sleep Restriction

Sleep Restriction is a procedure developed by Arthur Spielman specifically to eliminate prolonged middle-of-the-night awakenings (Stanford Medicine, 2023). The goal is not to restrict sleep but rather to restrict the time you spend in bed not sleeping. Sleep restriction starts by tracking how much time you spend sleeping in one week. Then, the following week, you are only allowed to spend that much time in bed. However, the time spent in bed should never be less than 5.5 hours. For example, if you go to bed at 10 p.m. and get out of bed at 6 a.m. but only spend 6 hours sleeping, you will be asked to only get into bed at 12 a.m. and wake up at 6 a.m. I know this sounds harsh, but within a couple of days, it will greatly reduce the time spent in bed, unable to fall asleep. The next step is to increase the time in bed by a couple of minutes, with the goal of still being asleep for all the time spent in bed but extending the time you spend sleeping. Eventually, you want to be in bed, asleep, for 8 hours a night. This procedure has shown great results for many people I know, and it is relatively easy to implement.

Sleep-Interfering Activation

This is a more general approach to sleep, and many of the techniques we already discussed in this book are also used within the sleep-interfering activation technique of CBT-I. This approach includes a variety of relaxation techniques, stress management skills, and reducing sleep-related worries. The goal is to shift the mindset from trying hard to sleep to allowing sleep to happen naturally. During sleep-interfering activation, you will use the hour before you go to bed to unwind and allow sleepiness to come to the surface naturally. This is usually when you do an activity that you find calming, like journaling or reading. Clock-watching isn't allowed during this process, so turn your clock away from you so that you don't end up spending time stressing about not falling asleep fast enough. It is also advised that you avoid exercising within four hours of your bedtime and that you should make sure that your sleep environment is one of comfort and calm (Stanford Medicine, 2023). As you can see, sleep-interfering activation basically focuses on your sleep hygiene and ensuring that you do everything you possibly can to improve your quality of sleep.

Foods and Substances

CBT-I also includes a process where you are instructed to remove certain foods and drinks from your sleep schedule, as well as look at certain eating habits that you might have. CBT-I helps you reprogram the way you view food and sleep. It encourages you to see them as two elements that work closely together, which is why you should manage your eating and drinking habits to ensure better quality sleep. During this section of CBT-I, you are encouraged to remove alcohol from your diet, even though it might speed up sleep onset and increase wakefulness in the second half of the night (Stanford Medicine, 2023). Another food or substance that you should avoid is caffeine. CBT-I highly encourages you not to have any caffeine after lunchtime to ensure that it's completely out of your system by the

176 | MAX SAMPSON

time you get to bed. Finally, this type of CBT-I focuses on eating habits and encourages you to eat big meals long before you go to bed since digestion can disrupt your sleep. Even when you are awake at night, resist the urge to have a midnight snack since that signals your body to be awake.

Biological Clock

The final part of CBT-I focuses on the biological clock in your body. It encourages people to connect with their biological clock and create their sleeping schedule around it. The goal is to align your bedtime and wake-up time with your circadian rhythm to ensure a natural energy boost as well as less difficulty falling asleep (Stanford Medicine, 2023). During this therapy, your therapist will help you understand your own biological clock, and if you are struggling to get aligned with your biological clock, they can prescribe medicine and other treatments to aid in your overall sleep well-being.

Cognitive Behavioral Therapy for Insomnia has many benefits, and it's a great place to start if you don't want to use medication. However, therapy and medication aren't mutually exclusive, and they can work together to your advantage. If you are struggling with your sleep, but you're not sure why, I highly suggest CBT-I treatment in order to get to the root of the problem and actually address the issue and not just the symptoms. If none of these treatment plans sound like something you want to embrace, there are still a few other treatment options that I'd like to share with you.

OTHER SUGGESTIONS

Let's say you've looked at all these treatments and advanced strategies, but you're just not sure whether you're ready for that type of treatment. What then? Well, don't worry, my friend, I still have a couple of tricks up my sleeve. In fact, there are five specific strategies that might help you fall asleep, which I would like to share with you now. These strategies are

- conducting a full-body scan
- changing your thoughts about sleeping
- performing recapitulation
- practicing silent chakra toning
- performing a sleeping mantra

Full-Body Scan

A full-body scan is one of my favorite ways of meditating. It's a simple pre-sleep meditation technique that allows you to become aware of every part of your body and let go of the stress that you might be holding in certain parts of your body. You can do a full-body scan by following these simple instructions:

- Start by finding a comfortable place to lie down with your eyes closed.
- Take a couple of deep breaths and relax your body with every exhale.
- Become aware of your body and notice the different sensations you are experiencing. Feel the weight, the temperature, and the positioning of your limbs and head.
- Focus on the crown of your head and relax your head as you breathe in and out. Slowly move down to your face and repeat.
- Move along your face, neck, and then your whole body, and notice any tension that you might be feeling.
- Exhale, let go of all the tension, and settle down to a stillness of sleep.

Changing Your Thoughts

When you struggle with your sleep, it can be hard to remain positive about it and not see it as a source of stress. Instead of viewing sleep as something you're struggling with, change your thoughts about it to something positive. See it as a period of rest where your body gets to restore, grow, and replenish energy. Don't simply view it as something that just happens or something that everyone should do; view it as something special that you get to do. View sleep as something sacred and not just something you're struggling to achieve (Brady, 2020).

Recapitulation

Recapitulation is the process of unpacking mental luggage from the day and cleaning out your mind in order to sleep. The goal is to detach from anything that happened in the last 24 hours and settle into deep sleep without carrying any stress or mental toxins (Brady, 2020). To perform a recapitulation, you can start by finding a quiet spot to sit or lie comfortably. Close your eyes and witness everything you did that day. In your mind's eye, go back to the first thing you remember about the day and then replay your day from that point of view. Watch your day unfold as if you were watching a movie. Don't become stuck in certain areas, though. The whole process should take about five minutes. Then, once you're complete, repeat the following words to yourself:

"Having witnessed this day, I release the events and images. They are now simply memories. I let go of everything and embrace peaceful sleep."

Silent Chakra Toning

If you're not familiar with chakras, don't worry, you can still participate. Chakras are the psycho-physiological energy that resides within the body. Every chakra is associated with a core physical and psychological need. However, our chakras can often go unbalanced during the day due to stress. So, in order to restore harmony between your mind and body, you need to tone your chakra by allowing your body to realign with your mind. This can be done through meditation or specific chakra exercises that you can find online.

Sleeping Mantra

The final card that I have up my sleeve is making use of a sleeping mantra. A sleeping mantra is a couple of words that you repeat to yourself in order to give your mind stillness and positive energy to focus on. It only requires one word that you repeat over and over again until you settle into a deep sleep. To perform a sleeping mantra, close your eyes as you lie in bed and softly or silently repeat to yourself, "Peace" or "Calm." Whatever word works for you and helps you find inner peace, continue to repeat the word until you fall into a deep sleep.

My friends, we're coming to the end of this magnificent journey, and I hope you've learned a lot of ways to ensure better sleep so far. However, before I send you on your way for some quality sleep, there is one more step that we need to take together on this journey, and that's the step of implementation. Yes, that's right! Everything you've learned so far needs to be put into practice if we want to see results, and that's exactly what the next chapter is about. So, grab a pen and paper because we're about to create your very own sleep diary.

8

YOUR SLEEP DIARY

Start right now with whatever you have. Six months from now it will be an absolute game-changing move in your life.

— HIRAL NAGDA

Before you start panicking and assuming that a sleep diary means turning into a teenage girl who writes down all her thoughts and dreams, take a deep breath. A sleep diary isn't a diary in the sense of writing down your deepest and darkest fears. It's more of a checklist, really. A sleep diary is a daily record of important sleep-related information that helps you track the quality of your sleep and build new habits (Suni, 2021b). A sleep diary can be as personalized as you want it to be, but usually, it includes things like

- time you went to bed
- what time you woke up
- how long it took to fall asleep
- exercise that day
- medications taken
- how many times you woken up during the night
- how many naps you took that day
- the perceived quality of your sleep

A sleep diary is an essential tool to evaluate your sleep journey and track your progress. It also makes it easier for healthcare providers to treat you since they can look in your diary for the necessary data required to diagnose you. A sleep diary is also a great tool to determine which habits might be negatively influencing your sleep and what you can do to improve the quality of your sleep. The best way to use a sleep diary is to keep track of it daily. Keeping a sleep diary will also help you to avoid any gaps in your memory about your sleep. If you're not quite up to updating your diary daily, try to update it at least once or twice a week.

In this chapter, we'll look at all the things to include in your sleep diary and how you can make the most of your sleep schedule.

SLEEP ENVIRONMENT CHECKLIST

The first thing a sleep diary will help you check is the quality of the environment that you might find yourself in. There are many factors that contribute to better sleep, but we're often unaware of the influence they have on us. It's almost like sleeping on a bulky mattress. It doesn't feel that bad until you visit a five-star hotel and sleep on a luxury mattress. Suddenly, your mattress back home doesn't seem so "fine" after all. That's why a checklist is a great way to make sure that everything in your environment is set up to promote quality sleep. Here's an example of a sleep environment checklist that you can use to determine the quality of your environment (Suni, 2021b).

Check ✓	Sleep Time	Notes
	Temperature set between 60° and 70°	
	No loud noises	
	Blackout curtains or a sleep mask	
	Clean and comfortable sheets	
	An inviting bed	
	Pleasant aroma in the room	

Start every nighttime routine by checking everything on the list for your ideal sleep environment to ensure a space that is welcoming, comforting, and welcomes sleepiness. You can also add other elements to your sleep environment list if you know that there are specific things that help you sleep better. For example, if you find a white noise machine helpful, you can add that to your checklist as well. Once you're finished with your sleep environment checklist, the next part of your sleep diary is to do a sleep hygiene check-in.

SLEEP HYGIENE CHECK-IN

A sleep diary can also help you ensure that your sleep hygiene is up to standard. When I was still struggling severely with my sleeping disorder, people would often ask me, "How's your sleep hygiene?" I would usually respond immediately with, "It's fine." However, looking back, I can now see that it was most definitely not the case. The truth is, I didn't know what good sleep hygiene was supposed to look like. That's where the sleep hygiene check-in comes in so handy. It helps us recognize what contributes to good sleep hygiene and objectively view our own sleep hygiene. Your sleep hygiene check-in should include the following questions (Suni, 2021b).

- Is my use of caffeine and alcohol affecting my sleep quality?
- Am I taking naps that are too long and often affect my nights?
- Do I feel rested in the morning, or do I feel drowsy?
- Is my sleep often disrupted at night?
- Am I allowing myself enough time to sleep?
- Is my sleep schedule consistent?
- Am I spending a lot of time in bed trying to fall asleep?

These questions serve as a wonderful reminder of what we can do personally to contribute to better sleep. There are many things that we can do to improve our sleep, even when we suffer from a sleeping disorder. However, we need to be intentional with our sleep hygiene and try our best to keep our habits and sleeping quality clean and highly effective. So, what's left to do? Once you've completed your sleep hygiene check-in and evaluated your sleep environment using the checklist provided, you can proceed with your sleep diary. As I mentioned earlier, you can customize your sleep diary however you want, but if you're not sure where to start, here's a template that you can use to get started.

188 | MAX SAMPSON

SLEEP DIARY TEMPLATE

You can either print this template for yourself or create your own. Whatever is easiest for you to stick with, do that. I want to challenge you to stick with a sleep diary for 21 days and see how it affects the quality of your sleep.

Morning							
Day of the week	Sun	Mon	Tue	Wed	Thur	Fri	Sat
What time did you get into bed?							
What time did you try to sleep?							
How long did it take?							
What time did you wake up?							
How many times did you wake up during the night?							
Number of times							
Number of minutes							
I slept a total of...							
How would you rate your sleep quality (1 to 5)?							
Was your sleep disturbed by anything?							

Evening							
Day of the week	Sun	Mon	Tue	Wed	Thur	Fri	Sat
I consumed caffeine in the morning (am), evening (pm), and late night (LN).							
AM, PM, LN							
How many cups?							
How much exercise did I get today?							
Number of minutes							
Time of the day							
How many naps did I take?							
How long was my nap?							
List of medications and supplements I took today							
Did I consume any of the following 2-3 hours before bed?							
Alcohol, water, milk, juice, a heavy meal, and caffeine.							

There you have it! Your very own sleep diary is ready to track your sleep and help you take your sleep quality to the next level. Remember, everything you've learned on this journey can help you, but not alone. It needs your application and determination! You need to commit to your sleep and make it a priority, regardless of what else is going on in your life. Sleep is and will always be essential for your survival, and if you want to live life to the fullest with joy and energy to embrace the things that you love, you need to prioritize your sleep first. Before I send you off to have the best night's sleep of your life, let's quickly recap everything we've learned so far and look at what our next steps should be. Remember, we're all different, and our sleep journeys might look completely opposite from one another, but that doesn't mean that we can't still help each other. You have everything you need to take the next steps on your sleeping journey, so don't wait a moment longer. Embrace this change and get excited about good-quality sleep.

Now That You're Rested and Energized...

A short review from you could make a world of difference to someone who feels like they will have to put up with poor sleep for the rest of their lives.

By giving your honest opinion of this book and sharing your insights on the 10-tactic path to restful slumber, you'll empower readers to wake up feeling like they should—refreshed and renewed.

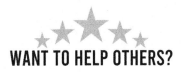

WANT TO HELP OTHERS?

Thanks for your support. My aim is to spark a sleep revolution that people of all ages can take part in. Sleep by night, and be your most alert, present self by day!

Scan this QR code to leave a review!

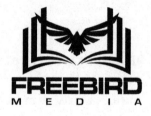

CONCLUSION

If there's one thing I know for certain, it is this: If I was able to conquer my sleeping problems and now wake up refreshed and excited for the day, then so can you! Do you remember that little boy I told you about at the beginning of the book? Yes, the one who didn't get invited to birthday sleepovers because of his snoring? Well, if that little dude was able to find a solution for his sleeping problem, then so can you. Why do I know that? Well, because you now have all the information you need to take your next step. Will it immediately be better? Probably not! But at least it's a step in the right direction. You don't have to be stuck in the mud anymore, desperately trying to find a solution. You have everything you need right in front of you. If you don't believe me, let's recap everything we learned on this journey and look back at just how much you've accomplished already:

- We started our journey together by looking at the importance of sleep. We discovered that sleep is essential, and we took a closer look at what happens within our brains and bodies when we go to sleep. This helped us identify the benefits of good sleep and debunk some old myths about sleep.
- Next, we learned about the different sleeping disorders. While there are many sleeping disorders that are all paralyzing in their own way, we learned that each one is different and has its own causes. We also looked at how sleeping disorders can lead to other mental health-related issues.
- In Chapter 3, we explored five lifestyle changes that we can all make to improve our sleep quality. While some of these lifestyle changes seem simple enough, we also learned that they require intentionality and effort.
- Together, we also looked at different types of medication that can be used to treat sleep disorders. Whether prescribed or over-the-counter, medication should be handled with care and respect. It's essential that you work

closely with your healthcare provider to ensure that you are using the right medication at the right dosage.

- If you're not quite ready for medications, in Chapter 5, we explored alternative treatments, which ranged from acupuncture to sleep hypnosis. Each treatment has its own pros and cons, so it's up to you to determine which type of treatment you're open to trying and which you're cautious of.

- Next, we looked at managing sleep disorders over the long term. It's not easy to live with a sleeping disorder, but it's also not impossible! When you are prepared, you can manage any sleep disorder over the long term.

- In Chapter 7, we looked at advanced strategies for better sleep, which included therapy as well as different medical devices. All in all, it showed us alternative strategies that we can implement to fight our sleeping disorders.

- Finally, we looked at why keeping a sleep diary is essential and how we can each create our own sleep diary template.

When we summarize all that we've learned so far, it's safe to assume that we all understand the importance of sleep. However, it's also clear that we now have what we need to take the next step. Whether that step is to go see a doctor or a specialist, or whether it is to seriously change some life habits, you know what you can do. You don't have to wait for a miracle solution anymore. You can take it into your own hands and do something about it. I hope that you are excited to embark on this sleeping journey and that you will experience the best night's sleep you've ever had tonight!

Remember, to sleep well is to live well, so don't waste any more time. Be kind to yourself and take a break when you need one. Just like everything else in life, this is a journey, and everything won't be moonshine and roses right away. Be patient, take a nap, and know that better-quality sleep is right around the corner.

If you enjoyed this book, it would mean the world to me if you could leave a review on Amazon. Or, better yet, pass along the book to someone else who can also make use of it. May you sleep like a baby tonight, waking up feeling refreshed and ready to tackle what-ever might come next. You've got this!

REFERENCES

7 Ways to Help A Friend With Sleep-Wake Disorder. (2022, May 26). The Recovery Village Drug and Alcohol Rehab. https://www.therecov eryvillage.com/mental-health/circadian-rhythm-sleep-wake-disor der/how-to-help-a-friend-with-sleep-wake-disorder/#:~:text=If% 20your%20loved%20one%20is

8 Ways Technology Can Help You Sleep Better. (2022, November 4). Alaska Sleep Clinic. https://www.alaskasleep.com/~alaskasl/8-ways-tech nology-can-help-you-sleep-better/#:~:text=Interior%20Light% 20Brightness%20Control&text=Using%20smart%20lightbulbs% 2C%20you%20can

Begum, J. (2023, May 2). *Alternative Treatments for Insomnia.* WebMD. https://www.webmd.com/sleep-disorders/alternative-treatments-for-insomnia

Benisek, A. (2007). *Sleep Apnea.* WebMD. https://www.webmd.com/ sleep-disorders/sleep-apnea/sleep-apnea

Boland, B. (2021, May 26). *The Potential Risks of Over-the-Counter Sleep Aids.* Banner Health. https://www.bannerhealth.com/healthcare blog/teach-me/are-over-the-counter-sleep-aids-risky

Brady, A. (2020, January 7). *8 Meditations and Mind-Body Practices to Help You Sleep.* Chopra. https://chopra.com/articles/8-meditations-and-mind-body-practices-to-help-you-sleep

Gallagher, A. (2021, October 27). *Eight benefits of a good night's sleep.* Bupa. https://www.bupa.co.uk/newsroom/ourviews/benefits-good-night-sleep

Gillette, H. (2023, January 27). *Is Chronic Insomnia Common?* Healthline. https://www.healthline.com/health/insomnia/how-common-is-insomnia

Gupta, S. (2023, January 27). *What Is Shift Work Sleep Disorder?* Verywell Mind. https://www.verywellmind.com/shift-work-sleep-disorder-7098445

Health Mythbusting: How Much Sleep Do We Really Need? (2023, May 25). Evidation. https://evidation.com/blog/health-mythbusting-how-much-sleep-do-we-really-need

Insomnia - Symptoms and causes. (2016). Mayo Clinic. https://www.mayoclinic.org/diseases-conditions/insomnia/symptoms-causes/syc-20355167

Insomnia. (2015). Cleveland Clinic. https://my.clevelandclinic.org/health/diseases/12119-insomnia

Kaufman, A. (2023, January 12). *How to fall asleep easier? Here's 5 tips to hit the pillow faster and wake up more refreshed.* USA TODAY. https://www.usatoday.com/story/life/2023/01/12/how-to-fall-asleep-easier/10839025002/

Lamoreux, K., & Raypole, C. (2022, January 19). *Everything You Need to Know About Insomnia.* Healthline. https://www.healthline.com/health/insomnia#types

Layla Sleep. (n.d.). 30 Of The Best Sleep Quotes. https://laylasleep.com/30-best-sleep-quotes/

Lui, J. (2022, September 1). *The surprising link between sleep, your bedtime and your heart health.* Health and Discovery. https://health.osu.edu/health/heart-and-vascular/how-sleep-affects-your-heart-health

Mansur, A., Castillo, P. R., Rocha Cabrero, F., & Bokhari, S. R. A. (2023). *Restless Legs Syndrome.* PubMed; StatPearls Publishing. https://www.ncbi.nlm.nih.gov/books/NBK430878/#:~:text=There%20are%20two%20types%20of

Marcin, A. (2015, June 10). *10 Things That Happen to Your Body When You Lose Sleep.* Healthline Media. https://www.healthline.com/health/healthy-sleep/what-happens-to-your-body-when-you-lose-sleep

Narcolepsy: Symptoms, Diagnosis, Treatment, Tips for Living with. (2020). Cleveland Clinic. https://my.clevelandclinic.org/health/diseases/12147-narcolepsy

Narcolepsy. (2023, January 20).. National Institute of Neurological Disorders and Stroke. https://www.ninds.nih.gov/health-information/disorders/narcolepsy#:~:text=What%20is%20narcolepsy%3F

Newman, T. (2020, August 24). *5 sleep myths: How much sleep do we need?*

Medical News Today. https://www.medicalnewstoday.com/arti
cles/medical-myths-how-much-sleep-do-we-need#1.-Everyone-
needs-8-hours

Newsom, R. (2020). *Depression and Sleep.* Sleep Foundation. https://
www.sleepfoundation.org/mental-health/depression-and-sleep

Nunez, K., & Lamoreux, K. (2020, July 20). *Why Do We Sleep?* Healthline. https://www.healthline.com/health/why-do-we-sleep#what-
happens-during-sleep

Okoye, A. (2017, May 22). *The benefits of exercise for sleep.* The Sleep
Doctor. https://thesleepdoctor.com/exercise/benefits-of-exercise-
for-sleep/

Ott, E. (2022, August 25). *Best Devices for Sleep Apnea: Here's What Works
in 2022.* CPAP. https://www.cpap.com/blog/best-devices-for-sleep-
apnea/

Pacheco, D. (2020a, November 18). *Light Therapy: Can Light Combat
Insomnia?* Sleep Foundation. https://www.sleepfoundation.org/
light-therapy

Pacheco, D. (2020b, December 4). *Sleep Medications: Over the Counter
Options.* Sleep Foundation. https://www.sleepfoundation.org/sleep-
aids/over-the-counter-sleep-aids

Pacheco, D. (2021, January 22). *Exercise and Sleep.* Sleep Foundation.
https://www.sleepfoundation.org/physical-activity/exercise-and-
sleep

Pacheco, D. (2022, April 1). *Diabetes and Sleep: Sleep Disturbances &
Coping.* Sleep Foundation. https://www.sleepfoundation.org/physi
cal-health/lack-of-sleep-and-diabetes

Relaxation techniques: Try these steps to reduce stress. (2017). Mayo Clinic.
https://www.mayoclinic.org/healthy-lifestyle/stress-management/
in-depth/relaxation-technique/art-20045368

Restless Legs Syndrome (RLS): Causes, Symptoms, Diagnosis. (2020). Cleveland Clinic. https://my.clevelandclinic.org/health/diseases/9497-
restless-legs-syndrome

Restless legs syndrome. (2023, May 10). NHS Inform. https://www.nhsin
form.scot/illnesses-and-conditions/brain-nerves-and-spinal-cord/
restless-legs-syndrome

Shaw, G. (2018, August 1). *Are drugstore sleep aids safe?* Harvard Health. https://www.health.harvard.edu/staying-healthy/are-drugstore-sleep-aids-safe

Single Care Team. (2021, March 25). *How much sleep does the average American get?* The Checkup. https://www.singlecare.com/blog/news/sleep-statistics/

Sleep apnea - Symptoms and causes. (2020, July 28). Mayo Clinic. https://www.mayoclinic.org/diseases-conditions/sleep-apnea/symptoms-causes/syc-20377631#:~:text=Sleep%20apnea%20is%20a%20potentially

Sleep hygiene tips. (2023). Headspace. https://www.headspace.com/sleep/sleep-hygiene

St Luke's Clinic. (2023). *Cognitive Behavioral Therapy for Insomnia.* Stlukesonline. https://www.stlukesonline.org/health-services/procedures/cognitive-behavioral-therapy-for-insomnia

Stimulus control. (2023). Stanford Health Care. https://stanfordhealthcare.org/medical-treatments/c/cognitive-behavioral-therapy-insomnia/procedures/stimulus-control.html

Stibich, M. (2021, July 20). *10 Benefits of a Good Night's Sleep.* Verywell Health https://www.verywellhealth.com/top-health-benefits-of-a-good-nights-sleep-2223766

Suni, E. (2020a, August 14). *What is Sleep Hygiene?* (N. Vyas, Ed.). Sleep Foundation. https://www.sleepfoundation.org/sleep-hygiene

Suni, E. (2020b, November 6). *Nutrition and Sleep: Diet's Effect on Sleep.* Sleep Foundation. https://www.sleepfoundation.org/nutrition

Suni, E. (2020c, December 4). *Sleeping Pills: Medications & Prescription Sleep Aids.* Sleep Foundation. https://www.sleepfoundation.org/sleep-aids/sleeping-pills

Suni, E. (2020d, December 10). *Anxiety and Sleep* (A. Dimitriu, Ed.). Sleep Foundation. https://www.sleepfoundation.org/mental-health/anxiety-and-sleep

Suni, E. (2021a, February 17). *Narcolepsy – Symptoms, Causes, Treatment.* Sleep Foundation. https://www.sleepfoundation.org/narcolepsy

Suni, E. (2021b, February 25). *Sleep Diary: How and Why You Should Keep*

One. Sleep Foundation. https://www.sleepfoundation.org/sleep-diary

Suni, E., & Callender, E. (2020, October 30). *What Happens When You Sleep: The Science of Sleep.* Sleep Foundation. https://www.sleepfoundation.org/how-sleep-works/what-happens-when-you-sleep

Susanne Reagan: Sleep & Narcolepsy Patient Story. (2023). Cleveland Clinic. https://my.clevelandclinic.org/patient-stories/38-sleeping-beauty-writes-her-own-fairytale

Theobald, M., & Chai, C. (2019, April 2). *What Happens When You Don't Sleep for Days.* Everyday Health. https://www.everydayhealth.com/conditions/what-happens-when-you-dont-sleep-days/

Travel and Sleep. (2021). American Thoracic Society. https://www.thoracic.org/patients/patient-resources/resources/travel-and-sleep.pdf

Watson, S. (2020a, May 8). *Sleep Specialists: When to See One and Where to Find Them.* Healthline. https://www.healthline.com/health/sleep/how-to-choose-a-sleep-specialist#types

Watson, S. (2020b, May 15). *11 Effects of Sleep Deprivation on Your Body.* Healthline. https://www.healthline.com/health/sleep-deprivation/effects-on-body#Causes-of-sleep-deprivation

Your guide to over-the-counter sleep aids. (2019). Mayo Clinic. https://www.mayoclinic.org/healthy-lifestyle/adult-health/in-depth/sleep-aids/art-20047860

Zwarensteyn, J. (2022, March 8). *Alternative Treatments for Insomnia and Sleep Disorders.* Sleep Advisor. https://www.sleepadvisor.org/sleep/disorder/insomnia/alternative-treatment/

Printed in Great Britain
by Amazon

30080177R00116